CARE FOR THE AGED
A Coursebook for Nursing Students

All rights reserved

Copyright @ 2021 by

Ashley A. Bangcola and
Laarni A. Caorong

Published by Lulu Press Inc.
United States of America
ISBN 978-1-329-89576-8

DEDICATION

To the elderly, who have weathered storms to guide us into an easier path

To students who continue to hold the umbrellas

To Allah (SWT), and the sunshine after the rain

ACKNOWLEDGEMENTS

By Ashley A. Bangcola

Writing a book is more difficult than I anticipated, but it is also far more rewarding than I could have imagined. Although I have published research articles and studies, publishing a complete study guide is a significant accomplishment. This book was created after hours of hard work compiling my study guides and materials, and it arose from a desire to make things easier for my students. I hope that this study guide will be useful to both my students and nursing students everywhere.

However, this labor of love would not have been completed if it had not been for specific people in my life who assisted me throughout this difficult process. I would like to thank my family members, particularly my husband, Alex P. Bangcola, for being a supportive presence in my life. Thank you for encouraging me to reach for greater heights. I would also like to thank my niece, Saliha Gianni Klien A. Paudac, for helping me with research during the writing and editing process. Thank you for keeping me organized and on track. I would also like to thank my two daughters, Ashyanna Alexine A. Bangcola and Adia Arianne A. Bangcola, for their perspectives, love, and support. In addition, I would like to express my gratitude to Yawman Book Publishing House for their assistance in publishing this book. Your hard work is greatly appreciated.

Finally, last but not least, I would like to thank the Almighty Creator, Ya' Allah (SWT), without whom nothing in this life would be possible.

ACKNOWLEDGEMENTS

By Laarni A. Caorong

At the outset, the pandemic has allowed people like me to venture on things I thought would only happen in my dreams of becoming an author. This book was developed to provide educational material to nursing students that they could use to study geriatric nursing. Several days and hours were devoted to compiling this book. A lot of time was spent researching, revising, and organizing the book until its fruition. I hope that through this compilation, studying gerontology nursing will be a lot easier for nursing students. Coming up with educational material is arduous, albeit fulfilling. It is such an honor to be contributing to the academe through this work.

This book would not have been accomplished without the much-appreciated effort of my co-author, Dr. Ashey A. Bangcola, a colleague, friend, and mentor. I would like to thank my family, friends, and colleagues. Thanks to my students, who have been my inspiration. Moreover, I would like to express my appreciation to Yawman Book Publishing House. for their help in publishing this book.

Above all, my deepest gratitude to our Creator Allah (subhannahu wa'ta ala) for this blessing. Alhamdulillahi Rabbil Alamin (All Praise belongs to Him).

TABLE OF CONTENTS

Copyright page..	ii
Dedication	iii
Acknowledgements..	iv
Table of Contents	vi
Introduction	vii
Chapter 1 Concepts, Principles, and Theories in the Care of Older Adults	1
Chapter 2: Nursing Care of the Older Adult in Wellness	11
Chapter 3: Nursing Care of Older adult in Chronic Illness	27
Chapter 4: Core Elements of Evidenced-based Gerontological Nursing.................	35
Chapter 5: Ethico-Legal Considerations in the Care of Older Adult	45
Chapter 6: Communication with Older Person	61
Chapter 7: Guidelines for Effective Communication	67
Chapter 8: Geriatric Health Care Team	73
Chapter 9: Research Agenda on Aging	79
Chapter 10: Trends/Issues and Challenges on the Care of Older Persons	89
Chapter 11: Advocacy Programs Relevant to the Care of Older Persons	101
Chapter 12: Grandparents as Treasure Chest of valuable History, Values, traditions Wisdom	109
Chapter 13: Telehealth/Telemedicine and Older Persons	115
Chapter 14: Entrepreneurial Opportunities	121
Notes	130

INTRODUCTION

The term "learning" has several connotations in common parlance, but it is important to emphasize that learning is a process, not a product. According to Ambrose, learning is something that students do for themselves rather than something done to them (2010). In the current situation, the students will embark on a new learning approach to gain knowledge in Geriatric Nursing Care. This will be accomplished by participating in a self-learning chapter.

This book covers the fundamental concepts, principles, and standards of working with older adult clients. Gerontology, also known as Geriatric Nursing, is a nursing specialty that focuses on the care of the elderly. Gerontological nursing, like other nursing specialties, necessitates an understanding of the physiological changes associated with aging, keen assessment and monitoring skills, extensive knowledge of aging conditions, care implementations, and comprehensive knowledge of established standards and principles of geriatric care. It includes instructional materials that are beneficial to both the instructor and the students to facilitate instruction and learning. The primary goal of this learning material is to serve as a resource for students learning geriatric nursing, assisting them in gaining a comprehensive understanding and skills in dealing with older adult clients.

Chapter 1
CONCEPTS, PRINCIPLES AND THEORIES IN THE CARE OF OLDER ADULTS

Overview

In this first chapter, we start by discovering several aging perspectives as well as the aging demography. By going through the chapter, you will also learn about the theories of aging and its implications in the nursing practice. Since physiological changes are inevitable in aging, you will also explore the changes older adults experience physiologically by reading this chapter.

Learning Objectives:

At the end of the learning activity, you will be able to:

1. Describe the global aging phenomenon and its implication to nursing practice
2. Understand the theories of aging
3. Enumerate the physiological changes of aging

Subject Matter

A. Perspective on Aging
B. Demography of Aging and Implications for Health and Nursing Care
 1. Global aging
 2. Aging in the Philippines
C. Impact of Aging Members in the Family
D. Theories of Aging and its Nursing Implications
E. Physiological Changes in Aging affecting various systems

CONCEPTS, PRINCIPLES AND THEORIES IN THE CARE OF OLDER ADULTS

A. PERSPECTIVE ON AGING

Aging is a natural process that begins at birth and ends at death. It can be defined as the sum of changes that normally occur in an organism over time. The process of aging is progressive. However, not all persons necessarily show signs of aging at the chronological age. At the biological level, aging results from the impact of the accumulation of a wide variety of molecular and cellular damage over time. This leads to a gradual decrease in physical and mental capacity, a growing risk of disease, and ultimately, death (WHO, 2018).

Beyond biological changes, aging is also associated with other life transitions such as retirement, relocation to more appropriate housing, and the death of friends and partners. In developing a public-health response to ageing, it is important to consider approaches that ameliorate the losses associated with older age and those that may reinforce recovery, adaptation, and psychosocial growth (WHO, 2018).

B. DEMOGRAPHY OF AGING

Key facts (Global Aging)

- Between 2015 and 2050, the proportion of the world's population over 60 years will nearly double from 12% to 22%.
- By 2020, the number of people aged 60 years and older will outnumber children younger than 5 years.
- In 2050, 80% of older people will be living in low- and middle-income countries.
- The pace of population ageing is much faster than in the past.
- All countries face major challenges to ensure that their health and social systems are ready to make the most of this demographic shift.
- People worldwide are living longer.
- Today, for the first time in history, most people can expect to live into their sixties and beyond. By 2050, the world's population aged 60 years and older is expected to total 2 billion, up from 900 million in 2015.

- Today, 125 million people are aged 80 years or older. By 2050, there will be almost this many (120 million) living in China alone, and 434 million people in this age group worldwide.
- By 2050, 80% of all older people will live in low- and middle-income countries[4]

Key Facts (Aging in the Philippines)

- The country consists of approximately 103 million inhabitants, with less than 5% of the population 65 years and older (Central Intelligence Agency, 2016).
- 60 years and older population of the Philippines is expected to increase by 4.2%, whereas the 80 years and older population is expected to increase by 0.4% from 2010 to 2030 (Help Age Global Network, 2017).
- The Philippines's population increased by over 35% over the last two decades with the older adult population (60 years and older) expected to overtake those aged 0–14 years old by 2065 (Help Age Global Network, 2017).
- Currently, life expectancy of Filipinos is 57.4 years for males and 63.2 years for females (Help Age Global Network, 2017)
- The improvement in life expectancy can be attributed to advances in public health in the Philippines, which have eradicated many of the diseases that once caused earlier mortality in Filipinos (Coscoluella & Faustino, 2014).

C. IMPACT OF AGING MEMBERS IN THE FAMILY

Caring for aging parents has multiple impacts on one's family life, including emotional, physical, financial, and structural effects.

Emotional Effects

- ✓ Guilt for not being able to do more for parents;
- ✓ Anger for having to set aside your own needs or shift your priorities;
- ✓ Fear and anxiety, including anticipatory grief and fear of financial strain.

Positive Emotional Effects

- ✓ Enrichment that comes with relationships between grandparents and grandchildren;
- ✓ Increased opportunity to pass on stories and knowledge to younger generations;
- ✓ Having a sense of being able to give back to parents and grandparents, resulting in a "greater connection" between family members

Financial Effects

- ✓ Caring for aging parents often means extra costs related to home health care, medical expenses not covered by insurance
- ✓ May necessitate extra time from work.

Structural Effects

- ✓ Shift in family structure and hierarchy related to [the] matriarch or patriarch no longer being in their role;
- ✓ This shift can cause guilt and stress, as family members work to find a place in the new family dynamic

Physical Effects

- ✓ Prioritizing parents' care may impact one's health
- ✓ Caregiving for a parent with dementia can cause chronic stress and illness.
- ✓ Time pressure might result in caregivers giving less attention to their children

Source: Makofsky (2012). How Does Caring for Aging Parents Affect Family Life?

D. THEORIES OF AGING

Most individuals will live to experience aging. Most people will experience age-related deterioration as life progresses. The process is unavoidable. Hence, it is of significance to understand the process. There are a number of theories about the mechanisms of age-related changes.

There are mainly two categories of modern biological theories of aging: Programmed and Damaged or Error Theories. The programmed theories indicate that aging follows a biological timetable. This means that the aging changes are regulated by the genes that affect the body systems responsible for maintenance, repair, and the body's defense responses. On the other hand, the damage or error theories imply environmental assaults to the living organisms. The occurrences induce cumulative damage at various levels as the cause of aging.

The Programmed Theory

1.) **Programmed Longevity**, which considers aging to be the result of a sequential switching on and off of certain genes, with senescence being defined as the time when age-associated deficits are manifested.

2.) **Endocrine Theory**, where biological clocks act through hormones to control the pace of aging.

3.) **Immunological Theory**, which states that the immune system is programmed to decline over time, leading to an increased vulnerability to infectious disease and thus ageing and death.

The Damage or Error Theory

1.) **Wear and tear theory**, where vital parts in our cells and tissues wear out resulting in aging.

2.) **Rate of living theory**, which supports the theory that the greater an organism's rate of oxygen basal, metabolism, the shorter its life span.

3.) **Cross-linking theory**, according to which an accumulation of cross-linked proteins damages cells and tissues, slowing down bodily processes and thus result in aging.

4.) **Free radicals' theory**, which proposes that superoxide and other free radicals cause damage to the macromolecular components of the cell, giving rise to accumulated damage causing cells, and eventually organs, to stop functioning.

Below is the summary of some of the commonly discussed theories and their relation to aging:

Disengagement Theory *(Chenbaum & Bengtson, 1994)*

- Refers to an inevitable process in which many of the relationships between a person and other members of society are severed & those remaining are altered in quality.
- Withdrawal may be initiated by the ageing person or by society, and may be partial or total.
- It was observed that older people are less involved with life than they were as younger adults.
- As people age, they experience greater distance from society & they develop new types of relationships with society.
- This theory is recognized as the first formal theory that attempted to explain the process of growing older.

Activity Theory *(Diggs, 2008)*

- Is another theory that describes the psychosocial aging process.
- Activity theory emphasizes the importance of ongoing social activity.
- This theory suggests that a person's self-concept is related to the roles held by that person i.e. retiring may not be so harmful if the person actively maintains other roles, such as familial roles, recreational roles, volunteer & community roles.
- To maintain a positive sense of self the person must substitute new roles for those that are lost because of age. And studies show that the type of activity does matter, just as it does with younger people.

The Free Radical Theory *(Harman, 1956)*

- The term free radical describes any molecule with a free electron, which makes it react with healthy molecules in a destructive way.
- Because the free radical molecule has an extra electron it creates an extra negative charge. This unbalanced energy makes the free radical bind itself to another balanced molecule as it tries to steal electrons. In

so doing, the balanced molecule becomes unbalanced and thus a free radical itself.
- It is known that diet, lifestyle, drugs (e.g., tobacco and alcohol) and radiation etc., are all accelerators of free radical production within the body.

The Membrane Theory of Aging *(Zs.-Nagy, 1994)*

A. According to this theory it is the age-related changes of the cell's ability to transfer chemicals, heat and electrical processes that impair it.
B. As we grow older the cell membrane becomes less lipid (less watery and more solid). This impedes its efficiency to conduct normal function and in particular, there is a toxic accumulation

E. PHYSIOLOGICAL CHANGES OF AGING

Changes	Health Promotion Strategies
Cardiovascular System Decreased cardiac output; diminished ability to respond to stress; heart rate and stroke volume do not increase with maximum demand; slower heart recovery rate; increased blood pressure; orthostatic hypotension	Exercise regularly; pace activities; avoid smoking; eat a low-fat, low salt diet; participate in stress-reduction activities; check blood pressure regularly; medication adherence; weight control; encourage slow rising from a resting position
Respiratory System Increase in residual lung volume; decrease in vital capacity; decrease gas exchange and diffusing capacity; decreased cough efficiency	Exercise regularly; avoid smoking; take adequate fluids to liquefy secretions; receive yearly influenza immunization; avoid exposure to upper respiratory tract infections
Integumentary System Decreased protection against trauma and sun exposure; decreased protection against temperature extremes; diminished secretion of natural oils and perspirations	Avoid solar exposure (clothing, sunscreen, stay indoor); dress properly for temperature; maintain a safe indoor temperature; shower preferably to tub bath; moisturize skin

Reproductive System Female: Vaginal narrowing and decreased elasticity; decreased vaginal secretions Male: Decreased size of penis and testes Male and Female: Slower sexual response	May require vaginal estrogen replacement; gynecology/urology follow-up; use a lubricant with intercourse
Musculoskeletal System Loss of bone density; loss of muscle strength and size; degenerated joint cartilage	Exercise regularly; eat a high-calcium diet; limit phosphorus intake; take calcium and vitamin D supplements as prescribed
Urinary System Male: Benign prostatic hyperplasia Female: Relaxed perineal muscles, detrusor instability (urge incontinence), urethral dysfunction (stress urinary incontinence)	Seek referral to urology specialist; have ready access to toilet; wear easily manipulated clothing; drink adequate fluids; avoid bladder irritants, such as caffeinated beverages, alcohol, artificial sweeteners; pelvic floor muscle exercises; biofeedback
Gastrointestinal System Decreases salivation; dysphagia; delayed esophageal and gastric emptying; reduced gastrointestinal motility	Use ice chips, mouthwash; brush, floss and massage gums daily; receive regular dental care; eat small, frequent meals; sit up and avoid heavy activity after eating; limit antacids; eat a high-fiber, low-fat diet; limit laxatives; toilet regularly; drink adequate fluids
Nervous system Reduced speed in nerve condition; increases confusion with physical illness and loss of environmental cues; reduced cerebral circulation	Pace teaching; with hospitalization, encourage visitors; enhance sensory stimulation; with sudden confusion, look for cause
Special Senses	

Vision: Diminished ability to focus on close objects; inability to tolerate glare; difficulty adjusting to changes of light intensity; decreased ability to distinguish colors	Wear eyeglasses, use sunglasses outdoors; avoid abrupt changes from dark to light; use adequate in door lighting with area light and night lights; use large-print books; use magnifier for reading; avoid night driving; use contrasting colors for coding; avoid glare of shiny surfaces and direct sunlight
Hearing: Decreased ability to hear high frequency sounds	Recommend a hearing examination; reduce background noise; face person; enunciate clearly; speak with a low-pitched voice; use nonverbal cues
Taste and Smell: Decreased ability to taste and smell	Encourage use of lemon, spices, herbs

Source: Brunner and Suddarth's Textbook of Medical-Surgical Nursing 11th ed., Lippincott Williams & Wilkins, 2007

SUMMARY: This learning chapter provided essential information on the perspectives and demography of the aging population, among other things. It has been concluded that the global growth in the number of older adults has substantial ramifications for families, nursing practice, and society as a whole. Additionally, learning about the theories of aging as well as the physiological changes that older persons go through helped to facilitate a better understanding of the older population as they go through aging changes.

Learning Activity: Reflect on the following questions and answer as honestly as you can.

1. Briefly describe the current aging phenomenon and express its implications to the nursing practice.
2. How are the theories of aging change your outlook on aging?

Guiding Question:

1. How do you see the aging phenomenon today? Do you find it concerning or not? Why?

2. Knowing that older adults experience physiological changes, what do you think are its implications in your nursing practice?

Chapter 2
NURSING CARE OF THE OLDER ADULT IN WELLNESS

Overview

The second chapter continues with a discussion of geriatric assessment. It is critical to build a systematic strategy to completing a full evaluation of older adult clients and to use the right geriatric assessment instruments to acquire valuable data that can be used to determine the client's health needs. Furthermore, completing assessments would be pointless if we could not figure out what activities and strategies to take. In addition, this chapter examines the implementations that are required to meet the needs of geriatric clients.

Learning Objectives

At the end of the learning activity, you will be able to:

1. Develop a systematic approach in conducting geriatric assessment
2. Use appropriate assessment tools and techniques in assessing older adults
3. Design a plan of care for older adult clientele

Subject Matter

A. Assessment
   1. Subjective
      a. Nursing History
      b. Functional Health Patterns

2. Objective Data
    a. Psychological Assessment
    b. Physical Assessment

B. Planning for Health Promotion, Health Maintenance and Home Health Consideration
    1. Planning for Successful Aging
    2. Home care and Hospice
    3. Community-based services
    4. Assisted living
    5. Special care units
    6. Geriatric units

C. Implementation
    1. Physical Care of Older Adults
        a. Aging Skin and Mucous Membranes
        b. Elimination
        c. Activity and Exercise

    2. Psycho-social care of Older Adults
        a. Cognition and Perception
        b. Engagement with Life
        c. Self-perception and Self-concept
        d. Coping and Stress
        e. Values and Beliefs
        f. Sexuality and Aging

NURSING CARE OF THE OLDER ADULT IN WELLNESS

A. ASSESSMENT

The geriatric assessment is a multidimensional, multidisciplinary assessment designed to evaluate an older person's functional ability, physical health, cognition and mental health, and socioenvironmental circumstances (Bassem, Kim & Higgins, 2011).

Obtaining Subjective Assessment Data		
Nursing History	Functional Health	Patterns
Obtain: Biographical Data History of Present Illness Past Medical History Family History Personal Situation Review of Systems	Functional Status refers to a person's ability to perform tasks that are required for living. The Geriatric Assessment begins with a review of two key divisions of functional ability: Activities of Daily Living (ADL) & Instrumental Activities of daily Living (IADL). *ADL are activities that a person performs daily (e.g. eating, dressing, bathing, transferring between bed and a chair, using the toilet, controlling bladder and bowel functions). *You may utilize the Katz Index of Independence in Activities of daily Living (Table 1).* *IADL are activities that are needed to live independently (e.g. doing	Obtain also the following: 1. Health-perception-health-management pattern 2. Nutritional-metabolic pattern 3. Elimination pattern 4. Activity and Exercise pattern 5. Sleep-Rest pattern 6. Cognitive-perceptual pattern 7. Self-perception Self-concept pattern 8. Role relationship pattern 9. Sexuality reproductive pattern 10. Coping-Stress-Tolerance pattern 11. Value-Belief pattern

| | housework, preparing meals, taking medications properly, managing finances, using a telephone). *You may use the Lawton Instrumental Activities of Daily Living Scale (Table 2).* | |

Table 1. KATZ INDEX OF INDEPENDENCE IN ACTIVITIES OF DAILY LIVING		
ACTIVITIES POINTS (1 OR 0)	**INDEPENDENCE: (1 POINT)** NO supervision, direction or personal assistance	**DEPENDENCE: (0 POINTS)** WITH supervision, direction, personal assistance or total care
BATHING POINTS:_____	**(1 POINT)** Bathes self completely or needs help in bathing only a single part of the body such as the back, genital area or disabled extremity.	**(0 POINTS)** Needs help with bathing more than one part of the body, getting in or out of the tub or shower. Requires total bathing.
DRESSING POINTS:_____	**(1 POINT)** Gets clothes from closets and drawers and puts on clothes and outer garments complete with fasteners. May have help tying shoes.	**(0 POINTS)** Needs help with dressing self or needs to be completely dressed.
TOILETING POINTS:_____	**(1 POINT)** Goes to toilet, gets on and off, arranges clothes, cleans genital area without help.	**(0 POINTS)** Needs help transferring to the toilet, cleaning self or uses bedpan or commode.

TRANSFERRING POINTS:_____	**(1 POINT)** Moves in and out of bed or chair unassisted. Mechanical transferring aides are acceptable.	**(0 POINTS)** Needs help in moving from bed to chair or requires a complete transfer.
CONTINENCE POINTS:_____	**(1 POINT)** Exercises complete self-control over urination and defecation.	**(0 POINTS)** Is partially or totally incontinent of bowel or bladder.
FEEDING POINTS:_____	**(1 POINT)** Gets food from plate into mouth without help. Preparation of food may be done by another person.	**(0 POINTS)** Needs partial or total help with feeding or requires parenteral feeding.

Table 2. LAWTON - BRODY INSTRUMENTAL ACTIVITIES OF DAILY LIVING SCALE (I.A.D.L.)			
Scoring: For each category, circle the item description that most closely resembles the client's highest functional level (either 0 or 1).			
A. Ability to Use Telephone		**E. Laundry**	
1. Operates telephone on own initiative-looks up and dials numbers, etc.	1	1. Does personal laundry completely	1
2. Dials a few well-known numbers	1	2. Launders small items-rinses stockings, etc.	1
3. Answers telephone but does not dial	1	3. All laundry must be done by others	0
4. Does not use telephone at all	0		
B. Shopping		**F. Mode of Transportation**	

1. Takes care of all shopping needs independently	1	1. Travels independently on public transportation or drives own car	1
2. Shops independently for small purchases	0	2. Arranges own travel via taxi, but does not otherwise use public transportation	1
3. Needs to be accompanied on any shopping trip	0	3. Travels on public transportation when accompanied by another	1
4. Completely unable to shop	0	4. Travel limited to taxi or automobile with assistance of another	0
		5. Does not travel at all	0
C. Food Preparation		**G. Responsibility for Own Medications**	
1. Plans, prepares and serves adequate meals independently	1	1. Is responsible for taking medication in correct dosages at correct time	1
2. Prepares adequate meals if supplied with ingredients	0	2. Takes responsibility if medication is prepared in advance in separate dosage	0
3. Heats, serves and prepares meals, or prepares meals, or prepares meals but does not maintain adequate diet	0	3. Is not capable of dispensing own medication	0
4. Needs to have meals prepared and served	0		
D. Housekeeping		**H. Ability to Handle Finances**	
1. Maintains house alone or with occasional assistance (e.g. "heavy work domestic help")	1	1. Manages financial matters independently(budgets, writes checks, pays rent, bills, goes to bank), collects and keeps track of income	1
2. Performs light daily tasks such as dishwashing, bed making	1	2. Manages day-to-day purchases, but needs help with banking, major purchases, etc.	1
3. Performs light daily tasks but cannot maintain	1		

acceptable level of cleanliness 4. Needs help with all home maintenance tasks 5. Does not participate in any housekeeping tasks	1 0	3. Incapable of handling money	0
Score		**Score**	
Total score_____ A summary score ranges from 0 (low function, dependent) to 8 (high function, independent) for women and 0 through 5 for men to avoid potential gender bias.			

OBTAINING OBJECTIVE ASSESSMENT DATA	
Physical Assessment	**Psychological Assessment**
Include the following: ✓ General Observation & Vital Signs ✓ Skin ✓ HEENT ✓ Cardiovascular ✓ Lungs ✓ Breast Exam ✓ Abdomen ✓ Extremities ✓ Rectal ✓ Pelvic Examination ✓ Neurological	*A psychological assessment evaluates thinking, learning and behavior.* You may use the following assessment tools to assess an older adult client: The Geriatric Depression Scale (Table 3) Short Confusion Assessment Method (Table 4) Mini-Mental State Examination (Table 5)

Table 3. GERIATRIC DEPRESSION SCALE

Instructions: Choose the best answer for how you felt over the past week.

No.	Question	Answer	Score
1.	Are you basically satisfied with your life?	YES / NO	
2.	Have you dropped many of your activities and interests?	YES / NO	
3.	Do you feel that your life is empty?	YES / NO	
4.	Do you often get bored?	YES / NO	
5.	Are you hopeful about the future?	YES / NO	
6.	Are you bothered by thoughts you can't get out of your head?	YES / NO	
7.	Are you in good spirits most of the time?	YES / NO	
8.	Are you afraid that something bad is going to happen to you?	YES / NO	
9.	Do you feel happy most of the time?	YES / NO	
10.	Do you often feel helpless?	YES / NO	
11.	Do you often get restless and fidgety?	YES / NO	
12.	Do you prefer to stay at home, rather than going out and doing new things?	YES / NO	
13.	Do you frequently worry about the future?	YES / NO	
14.	Do you feel you have more problems with memory than most?	YES / NO	
15.	Do you think it is wonderful to be alive now?	YES / NO	
16.	Do you often feel downhearted and blue?	YES / NO	
17.	Do you feel pretty worthless the way you are now?	YES / NO	
18.	Do you worry a lot about the past?	YES / NO	

19.	Do you find life very exciting?	YES / NO	
20.	Is it hard for you to get started on new projects?	YES / NO	
21.	Do you feel full of energy?	YES / NO	
22.	Do you feel that your situation is hopeless?	YES / NO	
23.	Do you think that most people are better off than you are?	YES / NO	
24.	Do you frequently get upset over little things?	YES / NO	
25.	Do you frequently feel like crying?	YES / NO	
26.	Do you have trouble concentrating?	YES / NO	
27.	Do you enjoy getting up in the morning?	YES / NO	
28.	Do you prefer to avoid social gatherings?	YES / NO	
29.	Is it easy for you to make decisions?	YES / NO	
30.	Is your mind as clear as it used to be?	YES / NO	
		TOTAL	

This is the original **scoring** for the scale: One point for each of these answers. Cutoff: normal-0-9; mild depressives-10-19; severe depressives-20-30.

1.	NO	6. YES	11. YES	16. YES	21. NO	26. YES
2.	YES	7. NO	12. YES	17. YES	22. YES	27. NO
3.	YES	8. YES	13. YES	18. YES	23. YES	28. YES
4.	YES	9. NO	14. YES	19. NO	24. YES	29. NO
5.	NO	10. YES	15. NO	20. YES	25. YES	30. NO

Yesavage JA, Brink TL, Rose TL, et al. Development and validation of a geriatric depression screening scale: a preliminary report. *J Psychiatr Res* 1983; 17:37-49.

Table 4. SHORT CONFUSION ASSESSMENT METHOD (SHORT CAM) WOR KSHEET

I. ACUTE ONSET AND FLUCTUATING COURSE
Box 1

a. Is there evidence of an acute change in mental status from the patient's base line? No ____ Yes ____

b. Did the (abnormal) behavior fluctuate the day, That is tend to come and go or increase and Decrease in severity? No ____ Yes ____

II. INATTENTION

Did the patient have difficulty focusing attention, For example, being easily distractible or having Difficulty keeping track of what was being said? No ____ Yes ____

III. DISORGANIZED THINKING   *Box 2*

Was the patient's thinking disorganized or incoherent, such as rambling or irrelevant conversation, unclear or illogical flow of ideas or unpredictable switching from subject to subject? No ____ Yes ____

IV. ALTERED LEVEL OF CONSCIOUSNESS

Overall, how would you rate the patient's level Of consciousness?

-- Alert (Normal)

-- Vigilant (hyper alert)
-- Lethargic (drowsy, easily aroused)
-- Stupor (difficult to arouse)
-- Coma (unarousable)

Yes ____

Do any checks appear on the box above? No ____

If Inattention and at least one other item in Box 1 are checked and at least one item in Box 2 is checked a diagnosis of delirium is suggested.

Confusion Assessment Method. Copyright 1988, 2003, Hospital Elder Life Program. Not to be reproduced without permission. Adapted from: Inouye SK, et al. Ann Intern Med.1990;113:941-8

Table 5. **SHORT PORTABLE MENTAL STATUS QUESTIONNAIRE (SPMSQ) version 1**

Question	Response	Incorrect Response
1. What is the date, month, and year?		
2. What is the day of the week?		
3. What is the name of this place?		
4. What is your phone number?		
5. How old are you?		
6. When were you born?		
7. Who is the current president?		
8. Who was the president before him?		
9. What was your mother's maiden name?		
10. Can you count backward from 20 by 3's?		

Scoring*

    0-2 errors: normal mental functioning

    3-4 errors: mild cognitive impairment

    5-7 errors: moderate cognitive impairment

    8 or more errors: severe cognitive impairment

NOTE ON SCORING

*One more error is allowed in the scoring if a patient has had a grade school education or less. One less error is allowed if the patient has had education beyond the high school level.

Source: Folstein, F. (1975). A short portable mental status questionnaire for the assessment of organic brain deficit in elderly patients. Journal of American Geriatrics Society. 23, 433-41.

B. **PLANNING FOR HEALTH PROMOTION, HEALTH MAINTENANCE & HOME HEALTH CONSIDERATION**

PLANNING FOR SUCCESSFUL AGING

What is Successful Aging?

Successful Aging is a term coined by Rowe and Khan (1996), who emphasized the interaction of three related elements including avoidance of physical illness and disability, maintenance of high physical and cognitive function, and continuing engagement in social and productive activities.

Tips for Successful Aging:

- ✓ See a physician when one feel ill.
- ✓ Take advantage of preventative care (vaccines, regular exams and standard diagnostic procedure e.g. mammograms, colonoscopies)
- ✓ Exercise, avoid a sedentary lifestyle
- ✓ Maintain good nutrition.
- ✓ Treat chronic pain
- ✓ Obtain adequate sleep.
- ✓ Think positively about yourself
- ✓ Build and maintain your social network

Source: Dr. Beata Chauhan (2016)

HEALTH SERVICES FOR OLDER ADULT CLIENTS

- **Home Care or Home Health Care** is a type of health service delivered in the home of a certain clientele. The client is visited by nurses, aides, and other health team members of the health team to aid and treat the client's illness, injury, or chronic condition.

- **Hospice Care** is a service designed to provide pain management, symptom control, psychosocial support, and spiritual care to clients and their families when the illness is incurable.

- **Community-based services** may be available for older adults to restore, maintain and promote independence, and support their physical, emotional and spiritual well-being. Such services may include transportation assistance, home repair & renovation, home health aide, medical visit, counseling, nursing visits, emergency response and therapeutic activities among others

- **Assisted living** is a type of living arrangement of which necessary assistance is provided to address the needs of older people.
  Types:

  a. *Group homes* are houses or apartments where two or more unrelated people live together.

  b. *Adult Foster Care Homes* generally provide room, board, and some help with activities of daily living. This is provided by the sponsoring family or other paid caregivers, who usually live on the premises.

  c. *Sheltered housing* is often in a home that offers personal-care support, housekeeping services, and meals.

  d. *Continuing-Care Retirement Communities*. These communities usually have various living options, ranging from apartments or condominiums to assisted living and skilled nursing home care.

  e. *Memory Care Assisted Living*. These are specialized assisted living facilities or homes that specialize in the care of older adults with dementia.

  Source: Assisted Living retrieved from
  https://www.healthinaging.org/

- **Special care units (SCU)** are a special type of facility that caters to older residents with special needs such as those with dementia or those with dementing illness. The care is provided by highly trained staff.

- **Geriatric unit** is a section in a hospital institution or facility that caters geriatric clients with varying health needs.

C. IMPLEMENTATION

Physical Care of Older Adults

Aging Skin	Prevent dry skin by limiting warm baths; limit use of harsh soaps to body surfaces; apply lotion or emollient to dry skin; drink enough water; eat a balanced diet especially food rich in protein; protect skin from harmful irritants
Elimination	Maintain bowel routines; encourage to decrease caffeine intake; increase fiber intake; increase fluid intake;
Activity and Exercise	Encourage to do regular exercise as tolerated such as walking, swimming; encourage to engage in social activities

Psycho-Social Care of Older Adults

Cognition & Perception	**Cognition** refers to the mental action or process of acquiring knowledge and understanding through thought, experience, and the senses. **Perception** is the organization, identification, and interpretation of sensory information to represent and understand the presented information. Frequently orient client to reality and surroundings; Reorient client to place, time & person; Enforce with positive feedback; Provide simple explanation; Observe client closely
Engagement with Life	An **engaged life** is living a life in a way that virtues and strengths are cultivated Encourage to engage and participate in fulfilling and productive activities; Promote social support; Promote leisure activities
Self-perception and Self-concept	**Self-perception** of aging is defined as a personal evaluation of one's own aging.

	Encourage to reflect upon one's life achievement; Encourage to do self-introspection
Coping and Stress	**Stress** is a state of mental tension and worry caused by problems surrounding life. **Coping** is the process of contending with life difficulties in an effort to overcome or work through them. Encourage to express feelings and emotions; Provide psychological support; Provide diversional activities; Promote relaxation techniques; instruct to avoid alcohol and caffeinated beverages; Promote exercise activity; Encourage deep breathing exercises; Encourage to meditate; Facilitate spiritual care
Values and Beliefs	**Values** are the motive behind purposeful action. A **belief** is an attitude that something is the case. Respect the client's religious beliefs; Respect client's decision personal preference and choices
Sexuality and Aging	Assess normal aging changes in terms of sexuality; Encourage to express concerns; Discuss worries and fears

Summary: Throughout this chapter, it was stressed that a full evaluation is essential in order to identify the health needs of older adult clients and to address their worries and challenges. Physical and psychological care for older adults with health concerns must be planned and implemented with meticulous subjective and objective health evaluations, helped by the use of suitable geriatric instruments, to provide the best possible outcomes.

Learning Activity: Reflect on the following question and answer as honestly as you can.

> Do you think using established geriatric assessment tools is important in assessing older clients?

Guiding Questions:

1. Create Nursing Care Plans. Your older adult clientele may be a family member or a relative. In this activity, you need to obtain subjective data by taking a nursing history, assessing your client's functional health and patterns. You also need to obtain objective data by doing physical assessment and use appropriate psychological assessment tool/s to assess your client's psychological status.
2. After completing your assessment, you have to come up with two Nursing Care Plans for your client.

Chapter 3
NURSING CARE OF OLDER ADULT IN CHRONIC ILLNESS

Overview

Chapter three discusses the persistent impairments and disorders that older persons have that affect their senses, cognition, and communication abilities. The sensory and cognitive changes that older adults go through might have a negative impact on their quality of life because they may have difficulty communicating and engaging with other people.

Learning Objectives

At the end of the learning activity, you will be able to:

1. Identify appropriate measures and care for older adults with chronic illness.
2. Recognize the unique health care needs of older clients with chronic health problems.

Subject Matter

A. Disturbance in Sensory
B. Chronic Confusion
C. Impaired verbal Communication

NURSING CARE OF OLDER ADULT IN CHRONIC ILLNESS

Chronic Illness has been defined as the irreversible presence, accumulation, or latency of disease states or impairments that involve the total human environment for supportive care and self-care, maintenance of function and prevention of further disability (Curtin & Lubkin, 1995).

Disorders experience by older adults are mostly chronic in nature which require treatment within a framework of changing lifestyles, adaptation to living situation, and attention to the person coping with the disorder (Burggraf & Barry, 1996).

A. DISTURBANCE IN SENSORY

Older adults experience changes in their senses (hearing, taste, smell, touch). The way their senses work is not as sharp as when they are still young. The sensory changes that older adult experience can affect their lifestyle as there may be problems in communicating, involving in activities and getting engaged with people.

	Alterations/Changes	**Disorders/Problems**
HEARING	Structures and functions inside the inner ear decline (the ear functions as an organ responsible for hearing and balance); Problem maintaining balance in sitting, standing and walking; Hearing loss (*presbycusis*); Inability to distinguish between certain sounds ~problems hearing conversations	<u>Presbycusis</u>-- problem maintaining balance in sitting, standing and walking; Hearing loss
VISION	Cornea becomes less sensitive; Pupils may react more slowly in	<u>Cataracts</u>-- clouding of the lens of the eye

	response to darkness or bright light; Lens become yellowed, less flexible and slightly cloudy; Eyes sink into their sockets; Eye muscles become less able to fully rotate the eye; Visual acuity declines hence the vision sharpness is altered; Difficulty focusing the eyes on close-up object (*presbyopia*) Reduced peripheral vision; Reading glasses, bifocal glasses, or contact lenses can help correct presbyopia; Keeping a red light on in darkened rooms, such as the hallway or bathroom, makes it easier to see than using a regular night light	Glaucoma -- rise in fluid pressure in the eye Macular degeneration -- disease in the macula (responsible for central vision) that causes vision loss Retinopathy -- disease in the retina often caused by diabetes or high blood pressure
TASTE & SMELL	In older adults, the number of taste buds decreases; The remaining taste bud also begins to shrink; Sensitivity to the five tastes often declines after age 60; The mouth produces less saliva as you age which can cause dry mouth, which can affect your sense of taste. The sense of smell can also diminish, especially after age 70. This may be related to a loss of nerve endings and less mucus production in the nose. Mucus helps odors stay in the nose long enough to be detected by the nerve endings	Decreased taste and smell can lessen the interest and enjoyment in eating. An older adult may not be able to sense certain dangers if he/she cannot smell odors such as natural gas or smoke from a fire.

TOUCH, VIBRATION, AND PAIN	The sense of touch makes one aware of pain, temperature, pressure, vibration, and body position. With aging, sensations may be reduced or changed. These changes can occur because of decreased blood flow to the nerve endings or to the spinal cord or brain.	The risk of injury from frostbite, hypothermia and burns is increased. Reduced ability to detect vibration, touch, and pressure increases the risk of injuries, including pressure ulcers.

Aging changes in the senses
US Online Library of Medicine, Medline Plus. Retrieved on August 13, 2020 from https://medlineplus.gov/ency/article/004013.htm

B. CHRONIC CONFUSION

Chronic Confusion is defined as an irreversible, long-standing, and/or progressive deterioration of intellect and personality characterized by decreased ability to interpret environmental stimuli, decreased capacity for intellectual thought processes, and manifested by disturbances of memory, orientation, and behavior (Gulanick & Myers, 2016).

Chronic vs. Acute Confusion	
DEMENTIA	**DELIRIUM**
• Chronic • Changes in mental abilities that occur slowly; over weeks to years • Caused by physical changes in the brain • Usually not reversible	• Acute • Changes in mental abilities that occur quickly; over hours to days • Caused by toxins in the brain • Usually, reversible
Sources: 10 Early Signs and Symptoms of Alzheimer's https://www.alz.org/alzhelmers-dementia/10_signs	

TYPES OF DEMENTIA	
Alzheimer's Disease	Progressive decline <u>May include problems with:</u> ✓ Memory loss (especially short-term) ✓ Executive function ✓ Personality changes ✓ Functional ability ✓ Sun downing ✓ Behavior ✓ Speaking and swallowing <u>Diagnosis</u> ✓ No single test to diagnose ✓ Mainly based on mental and behavioral changes ✓ Blood test and scans to rule out other causes <u>Treatment</u> ✓ No cure ✓ Some medications available to slow progression of symptoms
Vascular Dementia	Caused by changes in the blood flow to the brain; Can have a slow or sudden onset; Similar changes in memory, language and motor abilities as in Alzheimer's Disease. <u>Diagnosis</u> ✓ Screening to identify mental and behavioral changes ✓ Sometimes changes in blood flow to the brain can be seen on CT scan or MRI <u>Treatment</u> ✓ "What's good for the heart is good for the brain" ✓ Manage blood pressure, blood sugar and cholesterol

Frontotemporal Dementia	Frontal and temporal lobes of the brain shrink which affects their functioning; Usually occurs between ages 35-75; May run in families; usually first changes are in language and behavior; Often causes socially inappropriate behavior.
Lewy Body Dementia	Caused by abnormal deposits in the brain called Lewy bodies; Early, well-formed visual hallucinations are common; Often develop Parkinson's-like movements (shuffling gait, hunched posture, rigid muscles); Usually less drastic fluctuations in memory and thinking than in Alzheimer's or vascular dementia.
Source: 10 Early Signs and Symptoms of Alzheimer's https://www.alz.org/alzheimers-dementia/10_signs	

C. IMPAIRED VERBAL COMMUNICATION

Communication is defined as the transmission of information, thoughts, and feelings to be well received or understood. For communication to be effective, there has to be a message sent that is understood. Now, this can be challenging for clients who may have cognitive deficits or those who may have other communication issues that may cause difficulty as well to the health providers.

Impaired verbal communication is not an uncommon phenomenon when relating to older adult clients. It mainly arises from neurological disturbances categorized into: (1) reception, (2) perception, and (3) articulation. *Reception* is compromised as anxiety is experienced, or it may arise from a specific disorder. *Perception* is altered caused by stroke, dementia, and delirium. *Articulation* is hampered by mechanical difficulties, such as destruction of the larynx, respiratory disease, dysarthria, and cerebral infarction with neuromuscular effects.

Specific Communication Difficulties	Description	Nursing Action
Anomia	Word retrieval difficulties during spontaneous speech and naming tasks	Use visual aids such as picture when communicating with the client; provide positive encouragement;
Aphasia	A communication disorder that can affect a person's ability to use and understand spoken or written words.	Talk as if the person understands; Treat the person as an adult, and avoid patronizing and childish phrases; Be patient, and allow plenty of time to communicate in a quite environment; Use simple statement and phrases when asking; Use visual cues, objects, pictures, gestures and touch
Dysarthria	Impairment in the ability to articulate words as the result of damage to the central or peripheral nervous system that affects the speech mechanism.	Pay attention to the client; Allow more time for conversation, and conduct conversation in a quiet place; be honest and let the client know when you have difficulty understanding; repeat the part of the message you did not understand so that client does not have to repeat the entire message; remember that dysarthria does not affect a person's intelligence.

Source: Gerontological Nursing & Healthy Aging, 2nd edition by Ebersole et. al (2005)

SUMMARY: The third chapter provided essential information on the changes older adults experience in later life. Among them, there are those who experience changes in their sensory function and cognition. Other older adults also experience aging changes which impair communication. Recognizing the changes older adults go through in late life is essential for health care providers to understand them better.

Learning Activity: Reflect on the following questions and answer as honestly as you can.

1. What do you think are the possible barriers in communicating with older adult clients?

2. How would you effectively communicate with older patients?

Case Study: Mrs. Chase, who had been a stroke patient for six years, was admitted to a Home for the Aged Facility by her son John. John has been caring for his 70-year-old mother for six years, but he now intends to travel abroad in search of a job. Mrs. Chase is wheelchair-bound due to left-sided paralysis. Her stroke has also made it difficult for her to articulate or express herself. Mrs. Chase was discovered to be forgetful a few years following her stroke. She has no recollection of recent events, such as the food she ate at her last meal. She also has a habit of forgetting whether or not she has already bathed. Because of Mr. Chase's healthcare requirements, John had no choice but to place her mother in the aged facility.

Guiding Questions:

1. Why do you think Mrs. Chase experienced changes in her physical function, cognition and in her communication?

2. What specific nursing actions do you plan to implement?

Chapter 4
CORE ELEMENTS OF EVIDENCED-BASED GERONTOLOGICAL NURSING PRACTICE

Overview

For gerontological nurses to be safe in health care delivery, core elements of evidenced-based standards and principles must be followed. Along with it, gerontological nurses must also possess certain established competencies to be effective and efficient in rendering health care services to older adult clients.

Learning Objectives

At the end of the learning activity, you will be able to:

1. Recognize the importance of safe nursing practice by adhering to standards and principle in the care of older adults
2. List the necessary competencies in gerontological nursing care practice
3. Identify issues and concerns in relation to the care of older persons

Subject Matter

      A. Standards
      B. Competencies
      C. Principle

CORE ELEMENTS OF EVIDENCED-BASED GERONTOLOGICAL NURSING PRACTICE

A. STANDARDS

(Adapted from Iowa Intervention Project 1992; CGNA Standards 1996; Gerontological Nursing Association (Ontario) 2004; American Nurses Association, 2001; The John A Hartford Foundation Institute for Geriatric Nursing, 2000).

Practice standards describe the appropriate therapeutic health promotion, prevention, maintenance, and rehabilitation or palliation activities of gerontological nurses to facilitate client health.

STANDARDS	DEFINITION
STANDARD I: PHYSIOLOGICAL HEALTH	Gerontological nurses assist clients to maintain homeostatic regulation through assessment and management of physiological care to minimize adverse events associated with medications, diagnostic or therapeutic procedures, nosocomial infections or environmental stressors.
STANDARD II: OPTIMIZING FUNCTIONAL HEALTH	Gerontological nurses promote older adults to optimize functional health that includes an integration of abilities that involve physical, cognitive, psychological, social, and spiritual status (AACN & Hartford, 2000).
STANDARD III: RESPONSIVE CARE	Gerontological nurses provide responsive care that facilitates and empowers client independence through life course changes. A responsive care approach recognizes that certain behaviors are not necessarily related solely to pathology, but instead may be related to circumstances within the physical or social environment surrounding well older persons and those with dementia, and maybe an expression of unmet need (Wiersman & Dupuis, 2007).
STANDARD IV: RELATIONSHIP CARE	Gerontological nurses develop and preserve therapeutic relationship care. Relationship-

	centered care is an approach that recognizes the importance and uniqueness of each health care participant's relationship with every other, and considers these relationships to be central in supporting high quality care, a high-quality work environment, and superior organizational performance (Saffron, Miller & Beckman, 2006).
STANDARD V: HEALTH SYSTEM	Gerontological nurses are aware of economic and political influences by providing or facilitating care that supports access to and benefit from the health care delivery system. Systems to support and sustain practice changes should be in place, including ongoing education, policies and procedures and job descriptions (Crandall, White, Schuldheis & Talerico, 2007).
STANDARD VI: SAFETY AND SECURITY	Gerontological nurses are responsible for assessing the client and the environment for hazards that threaten safety, as well as planning and intervening appropriately to maintain a safe environment (Potter & Perry, 2009).

Source: https://pdf4pro.com/view/gerontological-nursing-competencies-and-standards-of-502188.html

B. COMPETENCIES

The American Association of Colleges of Nursing and the John A. Hartford Foundation Institute for Geriatric Nursing have worked in collaboration to develop the following competencies and curricular guidelines for geriatric nursing care to provide high-quality care to older adults and their families:

1. Recognize one's own and others' attitudes, values, and expectations about aging and their impact on care of older adults and their families.
2. Adopt the concept of individualized care as the standard of practice with older adults.
3. Communicate effectively, respectfully, and compassionately with older adults and their families.
4. Recognize that sensation and perception in older adults are mediated by functional, physical, cognitive, psychological, and social changes common in old age.

5. Incorporate valid and reliable tools into daily practice to assess the functional, physical, cognitive, psychological, social, and spiritual status of older adults.
6. Assess older adults' living environment with special awareness of the functional, physical, cognitive, psychological, and social changes common in old age.
7. Analyze the effectiveness of community resources in assisting older adults and their families to retain personal goals, maximize function, maintain independence, and live in the least restrictive environment.
8. Assess family knowledge of skills necessary to deliver care to older adults.
9. Adapt technical skills to meet the functional, physical, cognitive, psychological, social, and endurance capacities of older adults.
10. Individualize care and prevent morbidity and mortality associated with the use of physical and chemical restraints in older adults.
11. Prevent or reduce common risk factors that contribute to functional decline, impaired quality of life, and excess disability in older adults.
12. Establish and follow standards of care to recognize and report elder mistreatment.
13. Apply evidence-based standards to screen, immunize, and promote healthy activities in older adults.
14. Recognize and manage geriatric syndromes common to older adults.
15. Recognize the complex interaction of acute and chronic co-morbid conditions common to older adults.
16. Use technology to enhance older adults' function, independence, and safety.
17. Facilitate communication as older adults' transition across and between home, hospital, and nursing home, with a particular focus on the use of technology.
18. Assist older adults, families, and caregivers to understand and balance "everyday" autonomy and safety decisions.
19. Apply ethical and legal principles to the complex issues that arise in care of older adults.
20. Appreciate the influence of attitudes, roles, language, culture, race, religion, gender, and lifestyle on how families and assistive personnel provide long-term care to older adults.
21. Evaluate differing international models of geriatric care.
22. Analyze the impact of an aging society on the health care system.

23. Evaluate the influence of payer systems on access, availability, and affordability of health care for older adults.
24. Contrast the opportunities and constraints of supportive living arrangements on the function and independence of older adults and on their families.
25. Recognize the benefits of interdisciplinary team participation in care of older adults.
26. Evaluate the utility of complementary and integrative health care practices on health promotion and symptom management for older adults.
27. Facilitate older adults' active participation in all aspects of their own health care.
28. Involve, educate, and when appropriate, supervise family, friends, and assistive personnel in implementing best practices for older adults.
29. Ensure quality of care commensurate with older adults' vulnerability and frequency and intensity of care needs.
30. Promote the desirability of quality end-of-life care for older adults, including pain and symptom management, as essential, desirable, and integral components of nursing practice.

C. PRINCIPLES

The Principles of Geriatric Care include the following:

1. Biopsychosocial approach: the integration of consideration of physical, psychological, and social factors in providing health care
2. Use of multidisciplinary teams
3. Importance of chronic illnesses and geriatric syndromes
4. Importance of showing respect to older patients
5. Goal of maximizing function awareness and sensitivity to sensory changes
6. Age-appropriate dosing and avoidance of interactions of multiple medications
7. Continuity of care through the different components of geriatric care:
    a. Geriatric primary care
    b. Geriatric acute care
    c. Geriatric long-term care
        Community based

-home care
-adult day care
-respite care
Residential Services
-assisted living, board & care, adult care or residential care
-nursing homes
-retirement communities
Geriatric managed care: integration of primary, acute, and long term care.

Additionally, the *Division of General Medicine and Geriatrics, Stanford University* has established the following Principles of Gerontological Care:

Principles of Gerontological Care	Description
1. Aging is not a disease	- Aging occurs at different rates between individuals, within individuals in different organ systems - Aging alone does not generally cause symptoms. - Aging increases susceptibility to many diseases and conditions - Aging people are heterogeneous- some are very healthy, some are very ill.
2. Medical conditions in geriatric patients are commonly chronic, multiple and multifactorial	- Older individuals commonly suffer multiple chronic conditions, making management complex and challenging. - Acute illness are superimposed on chronic conditions and their management. - Treatment for one chronic or acute illness can influence the management of other underlying conditions. - Multiple factors are generally involved in the pathogenesis of geriatric conditions.
3. Reversible and treatable conditions are often under-diagnosed	- Older individuals, caregivers, and health professionals mistakenly attribute symptoms to 'old age'.

	and under treated in geriatric patients	• Many conditions present atypically in the geriatric population. • Systematic screening for common geriatric conditions can help avoid undiagnosed, treatable conditions. • Geriatric "syndromes" are commonly undiagnosed and therefore not managed optimally, such as; delirium, gait, instability and falls, urinary incontinence, pain, and malnutrition.
4.	Functional ability and quality of life are critical outcomes in the geriatric population	• Functional capacity, in combination with social supports, is critical in determining living situation and overall quality of life. • Small changes in functional capability (e.g., the ability to transfer) can make a critical difference for quality of life of older patients and their caregivers. • Standard tools can be used to measure basic and instrumental activities of daily living and overall quality of life.
5.	Social history, social support, and patient preferences are essential aspects of managing geriatric patients	• Understanding the patient's life history and preferences for care are critical. • Living circumstances are critical to managing frail older patients. • Caregiver availability, health, and resources are critical determinants of care planning for frail older patients.
6.	Geriatric care is multidisciplinary	• Interdisciplinary respect, collaboration, and communication are essential in the care of geriatric patients and their caregivers. • Various disciplines play an important role in geriatric care, e.g. nursing, rehabilitation therapists, dieticians, pharmacists, social workers, etc.
7.	Cognitive and affective disorders are prevalent and commonly	• Aging is associated with changes in cognitive function.

	undiagnosed at early stages	• Common causes of cognitive impairment include delirium, Alzheimer's disease, and multi-infarct dementia. • Geriatric depression is often undiagnosed. • Screening tools for delirium, dementia, and depression should be used routinely.
8.	Iatrogenic illness are common and many are preventable	• Polypharmacy, adverse drug reactions, drug-disease interactions, drug-drug interactions, inappropriate medications are common.
9.	Geriatric care is provided in a variety of settings ranging from the home to long-term care institutions	• There are specific definitions and criteria for admission to different types of care settings. • Funding for care in different settings varies and depends on many factors. • Transitions between care settings must be coordinated in order to avoid unnecessary duplication, medical errors, and patient injuries. • Integrate, multi-level systems provide the most coordinated care for complex geriatric patients.
10.	Ethical issues and end-of-life care are critical aspects of the practice of geriatrics	• Ethical issues arise almost every day in geriatric care. • Advance directives are critical for preventing some ethical dilemmas. • Principles of palliative care and end-of-life care are essential for high quality geriatric care.
Source: Division of General Medicine and Geriatrics, Stanford University https://geriatrics.stanford.edu/		

SUMMARY: Standards and principles must be followed in the practice of gerontology or geriatric nursing, as clearly stated in this chapter. The geriatric care standards and principles would serve as the foundation and guidelines for geriatric care practitioners to make their actions and decisions safe for the recipients of their care. Following standards and guidelines in geriatric nursing practice ensures that older adult clients receive safe and effective care. Furthermore, gerontology nurses must have certain established competencies in order to provide effective care to older adults.

Learning Activity: Reflect on the following questions and answer as honestly as you can.

1. What is the essence of following standards in nursing practice in the care of older adults?
2. From the list of competencies for safe geriatric nursing practice, list 10 competencies and identify weather you already possessed them or not.

Chapter 5
ETHICO-LEGAL CONSIDERATIONS IN THE CARE OF OLDER ADULT

Overview

Providing care to elderly people is not as straightforward as it may appear. Nurses must acquire the required competences to deliver efficient and effective health care to their clients who are older adults. Additionally, there are standards and principles that must be observed when providing care. Additionally, nurses must adhere to certain ethical and legal aspects of treatment. As a result, geriatric nursing practice is never as easy as one might believe.

Learning Objectives

At the end of the learning activity, you will be able to:
1. Describe the ethical and legal aspects involved in the care of older adults.
2. List the significant laws affecting the senior citizens of the Philippines.
3. Express understanding of the ethical considerations in geriatric care.

Subject Matter

A. Laws affecting Senior Citizens (RA 7432; RA 9257; RA 9994)
B. Medications of Older Adults (Polypharmacy)
C. Ethical Principles
D. Long-Term Care
E. Palliative Care

F. Advance Directives/DNR
G. End-of-Life Care
H. Spirituality among Older Persons
I. Ethical Dilemmas

ETHICO-LEGAL CONSIDERATIONS IN THE CARE OF OLDER ADULT

A. LAWS AFFECTING SENIOR CITIZENS (RA 7432, RA 9257, RA 9994)

RA 7432
An act to maximize the contribution of senior citizens to nation building, grant benefits and special privileges and for other purposes.
This act was approved on April 23, 1992.

RA 9257
Implementing rules and regulations of Republic Act no. 9994, also known as the "Expanded Senior Citizens Act of 2010," an act granting additional benefits and privileges to senior citizens, further amending Republic Act no. 7432 of 1992 as amended by Republic Act no. 9257 of 2003

RA 9994
An act granting additional benefits and privileges to senior citizens, further amending Republic Act no. 7432, as amended, otherwise known as "an act to maximize the contribution of senior citizens to nation building, grant benefits and special privileges and for other purposes.
This act was approved in the year 2010.

REPUBLIC ACT NO. 9994	
This Act shall serve the following objectives:	✓ To recognize the rights of senior citizens to take their proper place in society and make it a concern of the family, community, and government; ✓ To give full support to the improvement of the total well-being of the elderly and their full participation in society, considering that senior citizens are integral part of Philippine society;

	✓ To motivate and encourage the senior citizens to contribute to nation building; ✓ To encourage their families and the communities they live with to reaffirm the valued Filipino tradition of caring for the senior citizens; ✓ To provide a comprehensive health care and rehabilitation system for disabled senior citizens to foster their capacity to attain a more meaningful and productive ageing; and ✓ To recognize the important role of the private sector in the improvement of the welfare of senior citizens and to actively seek their partnership
Definition of Terms	*Senior citizen* or *elderly* refers to any resident citizen of the Philippines at least sixty (60) years old; *Geriatrics* refer to the branch of medical science devoted to the study of the biological and physical changes and the diseases of old age; *Lodging establishment* refers to a building, edifice, structure, apartment or house including tourist inn, apartelle, motorist hotel, and pension house engaged in catering, leasing or providing facilities to transients, tourists or travelers; *Medical Services* refer to hospital services, professional services of physicians and other health care professionals and diagnostics and laboratory tests that the necessary for the diagnosis or treatment of an illness or injury; *Dental services* to oral examination, cleaning, permanent and temporary filling, extractions and gum treatments, restoration, replacement or repositioning of teeth, or alteration of the alveolar or periodontium process of the maxilla and the mandible that are necessary for the diagnosis or treatment of an illness or injury; *Nearest surviving relative* refers to the legal spouse who survives the deceased senior citizen: Provided, that where

	no spouse survives the decedent, this shall be limited to relatives in the following order of degree of kinship: children, parents, siblings, grandparents, grandchildren, uncles and aunts; *Home health care service* refers to health or supportive care provided to the senior citizen patient at home by licensed health care professionals to include, but not limited to, physicians, nurses, midwives, physical therapist and caregivers; and *Indigent senior citizen,* refers to any elderly who is frail, sickly or with disability, and without pension or permanent source of income, compensation or financial assistance from his/her relatives to support his/her basic needs, as determined by the Department of Social Welfare and development (DSWD) in consultation with the National Coordinating and Monitoring Board."

The senior citizens shall be entitled to the following:	1. The grant of twenty percent (20%) discount and exemption from the value-added tax (VAT), if applicable, on the sale of the following goods and services from all establishments, for the exclusive use and enjoyment or availment of the senior citizen;
	   a. on the purchase of medicines, including the purchase of influenza and pnuemococcal vaccines, and such other essential medical supplies, accessories and equipment to be determined by the Department of Health (DOH).
	   b. On the professional fees of attending physician/s in all private hospitals, medical facilities, outpatient clinics and home health care services;
	   c. On the professional fees of licensed professional health providing home health care services as endorsed by private hospitals or employed through home health care employment agencies;
	   d. On medical and dental services, diagnostic and laboratory fees in all private hospitals, medical facilities, outpatient clinics, and home health care services;

e. In actual fare for land transportation travel in public utility buses (PUBs), public utility jeepneys (PUJs), taxis, Asian utility vehicles (AUVs), shuttle services and public railways, including Light Rail Transit (LRT), Mass Rail Transit (MRT), and Philippine National Railways (PNR);
f. In actual transportation fare for domestic air transport services and sea shipping vessels and the like, based on the actual fare and advanced booking;
g. On the utilization of services in hotels and similar lodging establishments, restaurants and recreation centers;
h. On admission fees charged by theaters, cinema houses and concert halls, circuses, leisure and amusement; and
i. On funeral and burial services for the death of senior citizens;

2. Exemption from the payment of individual income taxes of senior citizens who are considered to be minimum wage earners in accordance with Republic Act No. 9504;
3. The grant of a minimum of five percent (5%) discount relative to the monthly utilization of water and electricity supplied by the public utilities: Provided, That the individual meters for the foregoing utilities are registered in the name of the senior citizen residing therein: Provided, further, That the monthly consumption does not exceed one hundred kilowatt hours (100 kWh) of electricity and thirty cubic meters (30 m3) of water: Provided, furthermore, That the privilege is granted per household regardless of the number of senior citizens residing therein;
4. Exemption from training fees for socioeconomic programs;
5. Free medical and dental services, diagnostic and laboratory fees such as, but not limited to, x-rays, computerized tomography scans and blood tests, in all

government facilities, subject to the guidelines to be issued by the DOH in coordination with the PhilHealth;
6. The DOH shall administer free vaccination against the influenza virus and pneumococcal disease for indigent senior citizen patients;
7. Educational assistance to senior citizens to pursue pot secondary, tertiary, post tertiary, vocational and technical education, as well as short-term courses for retooling in both public and private schools through provision of scholarships, grants, financial aids, subsides and other incentives to qualified senior citizens, including support for books, learning materials, and uniform allowances, to the extent feasible: Provided, that senior citizens shall meet minimum admission requirements;
8. To the extent practicable and feasible, the continuance of the same benefits and privileges given by the Government Service Insurance System (GSIS), the Social Security System (SSS) and the PAG-IBIG, as the case may be, as are enjoyed by those in actual service;
9. Retirement benefits of retirees from both the government and the private sector shall be regularly reviewed to ensure their continuing responsiveness and sustainability, and to the extent practicable and feasible, shall be upgraded to be at par with the current scale enjoyed by those in actual service;
10. To the extent possible, the government may grant special discounts in special programs for senior citizens on purchase of basic commodities, subject to the guidelines to be issued for the purpose by the Department of Trade and Industry (DTI) and the Department of Agriculture (DA);
11. Provision of express lanes for senior citizens in all commercial and government establishments; in the absence thereof, priority shall be given to them; and
12. Death benefit assistance of a minimum of Two thousand pesos (Php2, 000.00) shall be given to the nearest surviving relative of a deceased senior citizen which

	amount shall be subject to adjustments due to inflation in accordance with the guidelines to be issued by the DSWD.
In the availment of the privileges mentioned above, the senior citizen, or his/her duly authorized representative, may submit as proof of his/her entitled thereto any of the following:	1. An identification card issued by the Office of the Senior Citizen Affairs (OSCA) of the place where the senior citizen resides: 2. The passport of the senior citizen concerned; and 3. Other documents that establish that the senior citizen is a citizen of the Republic and is at least sixty (60) years of age as further provided in the implementing rules and regulations.
The government shall provide:	
Employment	Senior citizens who have the capacity and desire to work, or be re-employed, shall be provided information and matching services to enable them to be productive members of society.
Education	The Department of Education (DepED), the Technical Education and Skills Development Authority (TESDA) and the Commission on Higher Education (CHED), in consultation with nongovernmental organizations (NGOs) and people's organizations (POs) for senior citizens, shall institute programs that will ensure access to formal and non-formal education.
Health	The DOH, in coordination with local government units (LGUs), NGOs and POs for senior citizens, shall institute a national health program and shall provide an integrated health service for senior citizens. It shall train community-based health workers among senior citizens and health personnel to specialize in the geriatric care and health problems of senior citizens.
Social Services	At least fifty percent (50%) discount shall be granted on the consumption of electricity, water, and telephone by the

	senior citizens center and residential care/group homes that are government-run or non-stock, non-profit domestic corporation organized and operated primarily for the purpose of promoting the well-being of abandoned, neglected, unattached, or homeless senior citizens, subject to the guidelines formulated by the DSWD. "Self and social enhancement services" which provide senior citizens opportunities for socializing, organizing, creative expression, and self-improvement; "After care and follow-up services" for citizens who are discharged from the homes or institutions for the aged, especially those who have problems of reintegration with family and community, wherein both the senior citizens and their families are provided with counseling; "Neighborhood support services" wherein the community or family members provide caregiving services to their frail, sick, or bedridden senior citizens; and "Substitute family care" in the form of residential care or group homes for the abandoned, neglected, unattached or homeless senior citizens and those incapables of self-care.
Housing	"The national government shall include in its national shelter program the special housing needs of senior citizens, such as establishment of housing units for the elderly.
Access to Public Transport	"The Department of Transportation and Communications (DOTC) shall develop a program to assist senior citizens to fully gain access to public transport facilities.
Incentive for Foster Care	"The government shall provide incentives to individuals or nongovernmental institution caring for or establishing homes, residential communities or retirement villages solely for, senior citizens
Additional Government Assistance	(1) Social Pension Indigent senior citizens shall be entitled to a monthly stipend amounting to Five hundred pesos (Php500.00) to augment the daily subsistence and other medical needs of senior

	citizens, subject to a review every two (2) years by Congress, in consultation with the DSWD. (2) Mandatory PhilHealth Coverage All indigent senior citizens shall be covered by the national health insurance program of PhilHealth. The LGUs where the indigent senior citizens resides shall allocate the necessary funds to ensure the enrollment of their indigent senior citizens in accordance with the pertinent laws and regulations. (3) Social Safety Nets Social safety assistance intended to cushion the effects of economics shocks, disasters and calamities shall be available for senior citizens. The social safety assistance which shall include, but not limited to, food, medicines, and financial assistance for domicile repair, shall be sourced from the disaster/calamity funds of LGUs where the senior citizens reside, subject to the guidelines to be issued by the DSWD."
The Office for Senior Citizens Affairs (OSCA).	There shall be established in all cities and municipalities an OSCA to be headed by a senior citizen who shall be appointed by the mayor for a term of three (3) years without reappointment but without prejudice to an extension if exigency so requires. Said appointee shall be chosen from a list of three (3) nominees as recommended by a general assembly of senior citizens organizations in the city or municipality.
Penalties	Any person who refuses to honor the senior citizen card issued by this the government or violates any provision of this Act shall suffer the following penalties: (a) For the first violation, imprisonment of not less than two (2) years but not more than six (6) years and a fine of not less than Fifty thousand pesos (Php50,000.00) but not exceeding One hundred thousand pesos (Php100,000.00);

(b) For any subsequent violation, imprisonment of not less than two (2) years but not more than six (6) years and a fine of not less than One Hundred thousand pesos (Php100,000.00) but not exceeding Two hundred thousand pesos (Php200,000.00); and

(c) Any person who abuses the privileges granted herein shall be punished with imprisonment of not less than six (6) months and a fine of not less than Fifty thousand pesos (Php50,000.00) but not more than One hundred thousand pesos (Php100,000.00).

"If the offender is a corporation, partnership, organization or any similar entity, the officials thereof directly involved such as the president, general manager, managing partner, or such other officer charged with the management of the business affairs shall be liable therefor.
"If the offender is an alien or a foreigner, he/she shall be deported immediately after service of sentence.

"Upon filing of an appropriate complaint, and after due notice and hearing, the proper authorities may also cause the cancellation or revocation of the business permit, permit to operate, franchise and other similar privileges granted to any person, establishment or business entity that fails to abide by the provisions of this Act."

B. **MEDICATIONS OF OLDER ADULTS (POLYPHARMACY)**

Polypharmacy is characterized as a patient's use of numerous drugs, with 5–10 medications being the standard limit (Geriatric Rehabilitation, 2019). Polypharmacy has been linked to getting older, having several diseases, and being disabled. Several variables contribute to the occurrence of polypharmacy, according to Maher & Hajjar (2014). Patients may require multiple medications to control their disease and maintain a high quality of life. However, if you're taking numerous medications, you're more prone to have drug interactions. Medicine interactions can boost or decrease the effectiveness of a drug.

Polypharmacy allows doctors to prescribe new medications to counteract the negative effects of another drug.

Polypharmacy is associated with negative consequences (Maher & Hajjar, 2014) including:

1. Increased Healthcare Costs
2. Adverse Drug Events
3. Drug-Interactions
4. Medication Non-adherence
5. Functional decline
6. Cognitive Impairment
7. Falls
8. Urinary Incontinence
9. Affect the patient's nutritional status

C. ETHICAL PRINCIPLES

Geriatrics is replete with ethical dilemmas. Ethics, or ethical care, is a framework or set of guidelines for deciding what is ethically good (right) or bad (wrong) (wrong). When there is disagreement over what is the "correct" thing to do, ethical issues arise (Kane, Ouslander, Abrass, Resnick, 2013). When a decision must be made on whether a medical intervention should be carried out or whether the intervention is ineffective or unfeasible, an ethical problem develops. Answering ethical dilemmas is not simple; it necessitates a complex blend of sentiments, opinions, and evidence-based data (Kane, Ouslander, Abrass, Resnick, 2013).

Ethical Principles in Caregiving

There are four ethical approaches to holistic senior care that are both practical and ethical:

1. Autonomy refers to a person's ability to control his or her own fate.
2. Beneficence means acting in the best interests of the patient rather than the healthcare providers.
3. The goal of nonmaleficence is to protect the patient's safety rather than to create harm.

4. Justice aims for a fair and equal distribution of rewards and liabilities.

A person may be at risk of neglect or abuse if any of these ethical norms are disregarded (Leuders, n.d.).

D. LONG-TERM CARE

Long-term care (LTC) encompasses a wide range of services aimed at compensating for functional loss caused by chronic disease or physical or mental incapacity over a long length of time (Feder, Komisar, & Niefeld, 2000). LTC varies in frequency and intensity according on the receivers' needs, and it can include both hands-on, direct care and general supervisory help. LTC provides assistance to older people in two areas: activities of daily living (ADLs) and instrumental activities of daily living (IADLs) (IADLs). Eating, bathing, dressing, getting into and out of bed or a chair, and using the bathroom are examples of ADLs. IADLs are additional chores that are required to preserve independence, such as meal preparation, medication management, grocery shopping, and transportation (Feder, Komisar, & Niefeld, 2000).

E. PALLIATIVE CARE

Palliative care is a type of medical treatment for those who are suffering from a terminal illness. This sort of treatment focuses on alleviating the illness's symptoms and stress. The purpose is to improve the patient's and family's quality of life (https://getpalliativecare.org/whatis/).

Palliative care is offered by a team of specially trained doctors, nurses, and other experts who collaborate with a patient's other clinicians to provide an additional layer of support. Palliative care is based on the patient's needs rather than their prognosis. It can be administered with curative treatment at any age and at any stage of a serious illness (https://getpalliativecare.org/whatis/).

F. ADVANCE DIRECTIVES/DNR

An *Advance Directive* is a document that a patient gives to his or her doctors and other healthcare providers, as well as his or her family and loved ones, outlining the type of care he or she prefers if he or she becomes unable to make medical decisions.

A *Living Will* is a legal document that specifies the type of medical treatment you prefer in specific circumstances. If you are terminally ill or permanently asleep and unable to express or transmit your medical wishes, it takes effect.

One sort of advance directive is a *Do Not Resuscitate (DNR)* order. This allows you to refuse cardiopulmonary resuscitation (CPR) or other therapies that would attempt to resuscitate you if your heart or breathing stopped.

Source: https://www.makatimed.net.ph/patient-and-visitor-guide/patient-references/advanced-directives

G. END-OF-LIFE CARE

End-of-life Care is the term used to describe the assistance and medical care provided during the time of death. Such care does not occur only in the moments before the heart stops beating and breathing stops. Older people frequently have one or more chronic illnesses and require extensive care in the days, weeks, and even months preceding death (Providing Care and Comfort at the End of Life, https://www.nia.nih.gov/health/providing-comfort-end-life).

There are several things that can be done to make a dying person more comfortable. Discomfort can be caused by a multitude of issues. Depending on the cause, there are things you or a healthcare expert can do. A dying individual, for example, may be uneasy because of:

- Pain (Administer pain medications as prescribed)
- Dyspnea (Elevate or raise head of bed as indicated, administer medication to help ease breathing as prescribed)
- Skin irritation (Apply lotion to dry skin, Turn the patient to sides to avoid pressure sores)
- Digestive problems e.g. nausea, vomiting, constipation & loss of appetite (Administer prescribed medication for specific digestive problem, Encourage to eat but do not force)
- Temperature sensitivity (In case of shivering- cover the patient with blanket/s)
- Fatigue (Keep activities simple, Conserve patient's energy by providing necessary assistance).

H. SPIRITUALITY AMONG OLDER

Gerontologists have recognized the importance of spirituality to the well-being of older persons over time. Spirituality is likewise difficult to identify and define. Spirituality is an interior experience for many people. Spirituality, according to Moberg (1971), is the fundamental value on which all other values are based, the major philosophy of life – religious, antireligious, or nonreligious – that drives a person's behavior, and the supernatural and nonmaterial components of human nature.

Spirituality is important to many people who want to live a long and healthy life. In fact, many people consider aging to be a spiritual experience (Moberg, 2001). In a study conducted by Harris and colleagues (2000), it was discovered that having a deep spiritual life in later life gives life significance. Furthermore, many researchers who study spirituality and aging have come to the conclusion that spirituality grows with age.

I. ETHICAL DILEMMAS

When there is no clear or distinct resolution to a problem or issue involving a decision about care, safety, health, or quality of life for an older person, an *ethical dilemma* arises. This can also happen when there is a clash of ideals among professionals, senior citizens, and their partners or families.

Guidelines for Decision Making in Ethical Dilemmas
(2002 Code of Ethics for Psychologists New Zealand)

a. Determine which topics and activities are ethically important.
b. Develop a different plan of action, preferably with the help of a professional colleague or supervisor.
c. Analyze the possible short-term, ongoing, and long-term risks and benefits for the individual(s) and/or group(s) engaged or expected to be affected for each identified course of action.
d. Apply the principle, values, and practice implications to each course of action in light of the identified risks and advantages, and choose the one that provides the best balance between them.

e. Accept responsibility for the consequences of the selected course of action by taking it.
f. Evaluate the repercussions of the action, correcting bad outcomes if possible, and re-engage in the decision-making process if the issue(s) originally recognized are not remedied.

SUMMARY: Caring for the elderly necessitates a number of considerations in order to respect their rights and dignity. When making choices and decisions in the delivery of care, health care workers must pay close attention. Established ethico-legal concepts, controlling legislation, and consideration of the older adult patients' decisions and choices must all guide health care providers' actions and judgements. To avoid inflicting injury on older individuals, care must be based on ethical and legal standards. When faced with ethical difficulties, health care workers must make decisions based on acknowledged and established criteria.

Learning Activity: Reflect on the following questions and answer as honestly as you can.

1. Observe your environment. Do you think that the senior citizens are aware of the established laws affecting them?
2. Are the senior citizens of this country enjoying the privileges that are designed for them to enjoy?
3. In the health care setting, do you think that the standards of care for older clients are being practiced?

Case Study 1: Mang Fidel recently celebrated his 60th birthday. He has no formal education and went to the OSCA to obtain a senior citizen's identification card. Mang Fidel is unaware of any existing legislation concerning elderly citizens, other than the fact that by obtaining a senior citizen's ID, he may be eligible for a 20% discount on medication and transportation. For his heart issue and diabetes, Mang Fidel has been prescribed five different drugs. His ambition to obtain a senior citizen's ID stems primarily from his medical condition.

Questions:

1. From the items in RA 9994, what do you think are the 10 most important items mang Fidel has to know?

2. Since Mang Fidel was prescribed several medications (Polypharmacy) for his ailments, what necessary health teachings should you provide him?

Case Study 2: Mina, a 78-year-old woman, was taken to the ICU with a serious illness. During her admittance, she gave her attending physician an advance directive stating that if her heart stopped, she should not be resuscitated (DNR). After a week, Mina's condition deteriorated, and she suffered a heart arrest. Mila's condition was revealed to her family. Mila had to be resuscitated and the family were vehement in their desire to have Mila resuscitated.

Questions

1. What should the nurse do when a patient has presented an advance directive and a DNR instruction and there are family interference pertaining to the advance directive?

2. As a nurse, how should you address Mila's family?

Chapter 6
COMMUNICATING WITH OLDER PERSON

Overview

Considering that old age is associated with a wide range of aging changes, dealing with older adult clients must adhere to a set of principles and norms. As a result, it is necessary to adopt effective communication. The fact that there are communication hurdles when talking with older individuals should be recognized by nurses as well. Impediments in the communication process might contribute to inefficient care delivery in some situations.

Learning Objectives

At the end of the learning activity, you will be able to:

1. Identify therapeutic communication techniques to utilize in communicating with older people.

2. Identify barriers when communicating with older adult clients.

Subject Matter

- A. Effective Communication
- B. Communication Barriers
- C. Guideline in Communicating with Older Adults
- D. Information Sharing
- E. Formal or Therapeutic Communication
- F. Informal or Social Communication

COMMUNICATING WITH OLDER PERSON

Communication is a difficult process in and of itself, and it can be made even more difficult by the passage of time. Sensory loss, memory decline, and delayed processing of information are all symptoms of the typical aging process that can interfere with communication in elderly people. Communication can be described as the process of delivering significant information to another person or group of people. Communication necessitates the presence of a sender, a message, and an intended recipient. When the receiver has grasped the meaning of the message sent by the sender, the process is considered to be complete.

A. <u>EFFECTIVIVE COMMUNICATION</u>

Effective communication is essential in meeting the health care needs of older adult clients because it results in practical benefits such as improved health outcomes and a stronger nurse-patient relationship.

The National Aging Institute has recommended the following tips for Improving Communication with Older Patients:

    a. Use the proper address format.
    b. Make older patients feel at ease.
    c. Take a few moments to build rapport
    d. Make an effort not to rush.
    e. Interrupting should be avoided.
    f. Make use of active listening skills
    g. Empathy should be demonstrated.
    h. Stay away from medical jargon.
    i. Take caution with language
    j. Make a list of key takeaways.
    k. Ensure comprehension
    l. Compensate for hearing impairment (use of hearing aids)
    m. Make up for visual impairment (allow proper lighting, wearing of eye glasses)

B. COMMUNICATION BARRIERS

Sometimes there are barriers in the communication process. Communication barriers are components or factors that obstruct the process of receiving and comprehending messages or information. When working with older adult clients, the following are the most common causes of communication barriers:

1. Age related changes

    ✓ Changes in hearing (hearing loss) and vision can affect communication

2. Disease and disability

    ✓ There are different illnesses and diseases that alter the ability of older people to communicate. Stroke, brain injury, lung disease & dementia may result to impaired communication. Loss of teeth also may impair speech.

3. Environmental Factors

    ✓ The physical and social environment may have some positive or negative influence or effect on the way older adults communicate. The health care settings may have direct influence on the quality and quantity of interactions. These factors may include noise, living situation that are not conducive to social interactions.

C. GUIDELINES IN COMMUNICATION WITH OLDER ADULTS

Communication Dos and Don'ts When Working with Older Adults	
Do's	Don'ts
Identify yourself.	Assume that the person knows who you are.
Address the person using the name he or she desires (e.g. Mrs. Garcia)	Use "baby talk" or patronizing names such as "sweetie" or "honey."
Speak clearly and slowly in a low tone of voice.	Shout.

Get to know the person.	Make generalizations about older people.
Listen empathetically.	Pay too much attention to tasks and forget the person.
Pay attention to body language (Yours and theirs).	Ignore non-verbal messages as insignificant.
Use touch appropriately and frequently.	Be afraid to use touch as a method of communication.

D. **INFORMATION SHARING (FRAMING THE MESSAGE)**

Verbal communication entails sending and receiving messages through the use of words. Some verbal communication is formal, structured, and precise, while others are casual, unstructured, and flexible. Formal or therapeutic communications have a distinct intent and goal. Informal or social conversations are more general and are used to socialize. Both have a place in the nursing profession. Nurses must be proficient in both formal and informal communication, and they must understand when and how to use each.

Nonverbal communication occurs without the use of words. Tone of voice, body language, gesture, facial expressions, eye contact, pace or speed of communication, time and timing, and touch are all examples of verbal communication. Nonverbal communication can help older adult clients understand information or messages more clearly and easily. It also decreases confusion, agitation, and anger while increasing cooperation.

E. **FORMAL OR THERAPEUTIC COMMUNICATION**

Therapeutic communication is a deliberate and conscious process of gathering information about a patient's overall health status and responding with verbal and nonverbal approaches that promote the patient's well-being or improve the patient's understanding of ongoing care. When performed by an experienced health professional, this type of communication appears effortless and natural, but it is a skill that takes time, effort, and practice to master. Effective verbal communication necessitates the ability to send and receive messages using a variety of techniques.

When communicating verbally, nurses should know as much as possible about the other person involved, whether in a formal or informal setting. The communication techniques and words used by a person are influenced by their age, marital status, cultural or ethnic orientation, educational background, interests, and ability to hear and see. As nurses, we must exercise caution in selecting words that the patient understands. Listening carefully to the patient's speech can provide information about the appropriate level of language.

Also, keep in mind that different words can mean different things to people of different generations or cultures. *Gay* can refer to being happy and lighthearted, or it can refer to a different way of life. *Cool* can refer to either a temperature or something extremely enjoyable. *Bread* can be something you eat or something you spend your money on. When choosing your words, consider the older patient's culture, ethnicity, experiences, and perspective.

F. INFORMAL OR SOCIAL COMMUNICATION

In nurse-patient communication, simple chitchat has a place. Nurses would know nothing about their patients if they just talked about health-related topics. Small talk, niceties, and discussions about the weather, a favorite television show, or the latest news can convey that the nurse considers the patient to be a genuine person, not just a patient. This is likewise true in the opposite direction. Older patients frequently inquire about the nurses who care for them, including the nurse's family, interests, vacations, and so on. This is especially true in long-term care institutions, where the nursing staff typically becomes the elderly person's new family. When talking with older patients, don't be afraid to be "human."

Be open and honest with your senior patients. Explain why you won't be able to visit so that patients don't take it personally and believe they've done anything wrong. Don't be scared to utilize comedy in the right context. "Laughter is the best medicine," as the saying goes, but it's a medicine that's all too often in short supply among the elderly. Choose the appropriate time and location. Make sure the jokes are culturally appropriate. Always remember that it's fine to laugh at oneself, but never at someone else. People do not lose their sense of humor as they age. A funny story or animation might make their day a little brighter.

Source: https://nursekey.com/communicating-with-older-adults/

SUMMARY

This chapter covered how to properly communicate with elderly individuals. To acquire information about their overall health status, it is vital to communicate effectively with older adult clients. In order to construct care plans to address patients' health needs, they must first gather the relevant information and data regarding their health problems. To better comprehend client needs, geriatric nurses must pay attention to nonverbal clues stated and seen by older clients during dialogue.

> **Learning Activity**: Reflect on the following questions and answer as honestly as you can.
>
> Do you think you have already developed effective communication skills? If not, what do you think should you improve on?

Guiding Question:

You shall interview your grandparent or an eldest closest living relative. Through questions, you are expected to accomplish a _process recording_. You can ask any questions to your elder client. Before the interview, you must ask your client's permission that your conversation will be recorded and analyzed. Transcriptions must be done after the interview. The content must be analyzed by identifying key statements that are _therapeutic_, _non-therapeutic_, _formal_ or _informal communication styles_.

[**Process Recording** are the written reports of verbal interactions with clients. They are verbatim accounts, written by the nurse or student as a tool for improving interpretation communication technique.]

Chapter 7
GUIDELINES FOR EFFECTIVE DOCUMENTATION

Overview

Documentation is vital for providing critical clinical information about each patient's diagnosis, treatment, and outcomes, as well as for communication among members of the health care team. Because this aspect of the job has so many ramifications, geriatric nurses must practice effective documentation. Client health status must be identified using concise, effective, and proper documentation as the foundation for treatment planning, execution, and evaluation.

Learning Objectives

At the end of the learning activity, you will be able to:

1. Determine the ways of effective documentation
2. List the methods and formats of proper documentation

Subject Matter

A. Important General Information About Documentation
B. Documentation Formats/ Systems
C. Concise Documentation
D. Effective Documentation

GUIDELINES FOR EFFECTIVE DOCUMENTATION

Documentation is anything written or printed that is relied on as a record of proof for authorized persons. Documentation and reporting in nursing are needed for continuity of care; it is also a legal requirement showing the nursing care performed or not performed by a nurse. Proper documentation is important in the health care industry. Its purpose is to serve as a legal document as evidence of care and treatment provision; it also serves as basis to identify health status of clients for care planning, implementation and evaluation. Through documentation, consistency of care is ensured as it provides necessary information for the health care team members. Other purposes of documentation include health audit, research, education, and reimbursement.

To guarantee that the health care needs of older adult clients receiving health care support are addressed, a care plan must be in place. Nurses' progress notes in patients' charts play an important role in evaluating and amending patient care plans. The wants and needs of their older adult clients must be met by health care providers, particularly gerontology nurses. The adjustments documented in the progress notes will determine whether or not this is possible.

A. IMPORTANT GENERAL INFORMATION ABOUT DOCUMENTATION

Documenting needs to be completed as soon as possible after an event or incident. Progress notes are legal documents and must be filled out in the following manner.

   a. Progress notes must be recorded in black ink and printed.
   b. No correction fluid (whiteout) can be used.
   c. A line must be drawn through any corrections, the correction initialed and the information rewritten.
   d. A line to the end of the page must be drawn where documenting does not use all the line space.
   e. All notes must be dated, including the time of the incident.
   f. All notes must be signed and include the compiler's printed name and status

Source: http://compliantlearningresources.com.au/network/lotus/files/2016/06/Documenting-Skills-in-Aged-Care-Progress-Notes.pdf

B. DOCUMENTATION FORMATS/SYSTEMS

1. Source – Oriented Record

The traditional client record. Each individual or department writes notes in their own section or sections of the client's chart. It is practical because care providers from various disciplines may simply access the forms on which to collect data, and the information can be traced. The source-oriented record has always included narrative charting.

2. Problem – Oriented Medical Record (POMR)

The Problem – Oriented Medical Record was stablished by Lawrence Weed. The data are arranged according to the problems the client has rather than the source of information. The Problem – Oriented Medical Record has four basic components:

a. Database – consists of all information about the client, nursing assessment, the physician's history, social & family data
b. Problem List – list of identified patient's problem/s; the list is continually updated as new problems are identified & others resolved
c. Plan of Care – care plans are generated by the person who lists the problems.
d. Progress Notes – chart entry made by all health professionals involved in a client's care; they all use the same type of sheet for notes.

Example: SOAP Format or SOAPIE and SOAPIER (S-Subjective, O-Objective, A-Assessment, P-Plan, I-Interventions, E-Evaluation R- Revision); PIE (Problem, Interventions, and Evaluation); Focus Charting (focus and progress notes are recorded; focused on the client's concerns); Computerized documentation (store client's using computers) (Nurseslabs, 2013).

C. CONCISE DOCUMENTATION

Concise Documentation means giving not too much, or too little, information. If too much information is given, it may obscure the main point of the note. If too little information is given, the client may not receive the correct care. This could cause suffering to the client or may lead to legal consequences.

a. The information included
b. The words used
c. The structure of both the sentences and information

If care staff document only by exception and record objectively, this is a good basis for keeping notes concise since they will be necessary and factual. Often fewer words can be used to get the same message across. Below are some examples of using one word instead of a phrase:

Common Phrase	Alternative Words
Kept an eye on/ watched over	Monitored, observed, supervised
Put client's legs/arm up	Raised, elevated
Make the swelling go down	Reduce, decrease, alleviate
Kept on/ over and over again	Continually, constantly
All the time/ a lot	Frequently, often, continually, constantly
Take off	Remove
Every now and again	Continuously, often, frequently
Looks the same as	Resembles
Spoke too quietly to be heard	Inaudible
Singing one minute then swearing the next	Alternatively singing and swearing
Going on about	Complaining
Put client's clothes on	Dressed
Pulls faces	Grimace

*Source:*http://compliantlearningresources.com.au/network/lotus/files/2016/06/Documenting-Skills-in-Aged-Care-Progress-Notes.pdf

D. EFFECTIVE DOCUMENTATION

The following are guidelines for good documentation and reporting:

1. Fact – information about clients and their care must be factual. A record should contain descriptive, objective information about what a nurse sees, hears, feels and smells
2. Accuracy – information must be accurate so that health team members have confidence in it
3. Completeness – the information within a record or a report should be complete, containing concise and thorough information about a client's care. Concise data are easy to understand
4. Currentness – ongoing decisions about care must be based on currently reported information. At the time of occurrence include the following:

   a. Vital signs
   b. Administration of medications and treatments
   c. Preparation of diagnostic tests or surgery
   d. Change in status
   e. Admission, transfer, discharge or death of a client
   f. Treatment for a sudden change in status

5. Organization – the nurse communicates in a logical format or order
6. Confidentiality – a confidential communication is information given by one person to another with trust and confidence that such information will not be disclosed (Nurseslabs, 2013).

SUMMARY: In the field of geriatric nursing, documentation has numerous implications. Continuity of care can be achieved by accurate documentation, which serves as a foundation for the next course of action by health care providers in dealing with geriatric clients. Geriatric nurses must also practice good documentation because it has legal ramifications. For documentation to be regarded effective, it must be succinct, accurate, complete, and well-organized.

> Learning Activity: Reflect on the following questions and answer as honestly as you can.
>
> 1. What do you think are the implications/ results of a poor documentation?
> 2. Which of the documentation formats/systems are you most comfortable to follow? Why?

Case Study: Mrs. Jane Santos, a sixty-year-old client, sought admission to the ER. For three days, she had trouble breathing, chest pain, and a persistent cough. She is currently febrile as well. Mrs. Santos' other assessment results, as well as the interventions first administered to her in the ER, were as follows:

Nasal flaring and use of accessory muscle noted	Instructed to maintain bed rest with toilet privileges
Admitted on August 20, 2020 at 9am	Provide comfort measures
Provided O2 inhalation at 2 liters/min; head of bed elevated	For Serum potassium determination
Diet: NPO when dyspneic	For ECG
On CBR with TP	Started venoclysis with D5 NM 1l @ 15 gtts/min
Medicated given: Salbutamol 1 neb stat, Paracetamol 500mg IVTT now.	Initial VS: T-38.9; P-75, R-25, BP-110/70
Provide TSB	For x-ray APL

Activity: Make a documentation of the data provided above by demonstrating two (2) different approaches to documentation: source-oriented approach and problem-oriented recording.

Chapter 8
GERIATRIC HEALTH CARE TEAM

Overview
Collaboration and team effort are necessary elements in providing effective care for older adult clients. The geriatric health care team comprises professionals with specific specialties crucial in addressing client issues and concerns.

Learning Objectives:
At the end of the learning activity, you will be able to:

1. Differentiate the roles and functions of the members of a geriatric health care team
2. Recognize the importance of collaboration in the care of older people with health needs

Subject Matter
    A. Gerontologist/Geriatrician
    B. Nurse Gerontologist
    C. Occupational Therapist
    D. Physical Therapist
    E. Speech Therapist
    F. Case Manager
    G. Family/ Significant Others
    H. Nursing and Interdisciplinary Team

GERIATRIC HEALTH CARE TEAM

A health care team can be defined as a group of professionals with special roles. In the care of older adult clients, geriatric health care team is necessary to address client's needs (Bakerjian, 2020).

Geriatric multidisciplinary teams are made up of practitioners from many disciplines who work together to provide coordinated, integrated care with shared resources and responsibilities. A structured geriatric multidisciplinary team is not required for all older patients. If patients have complicated medical, psychologic, or social needs, however, such teams are more effective than practitioners working alone in assessing patient needs and developing an appropriate care plan. Management by a geriatrician or geriatric nurse practitioner, or a primary care physician, nurse practitioner, or physician assistant with experience and interest in geriatric medicine, provides an alternative if interdisciplinary care is not available.

The following are the goals of interdisciplinary teams (Bakerjian, 2020):

a. That patients can move securely and readily from one care environment to another, and from one practitioner to another.
b. That each problem is treated by the most qualified practitioner.
c. The care or level of attention is not duplicated.
d. The care is a comprehensive service.

Interdisciplinary teams must interact openly, freely, and on a frequent basis in order to design, monitor, or update the care plan. Members of the core team must work together and coordinate the care plan with trust and respect for the contributions of others (e.g., by delegating, sharing accountability, jointly implementing it).

Team members may work in the same location, allowing for informal and quick contact. However, with the rising use of technology (such as cell phones, laptops, the internet, and telehealth), it is not uncommon for team members to operate at separate locations and communicate using multiple technologies.

Physicians, nurses, nurse practitioners, physician assistants, pharmacists, social workers, psychologists, and, on rare occasions, a dentist, dietician, physical and occupational therapists, an ethicist, or a palliative care or hospice physician are all part of a team. Geriatric medical knowledge, acquaintance with the patient, commitment to the team approach, and effective communication skills are all required of team members (Bakerjian, 2020).

Teams require a defined framework to function efficiently. Teams should create a shared vision of care, specify patient-centered targets and deadlines, hold regular meetings (to review team structure, process, and communication), and track their success on a regular basis (using quality improvement measures). In general, team leadership should rotate depending on the patient's needs; the patient's progress should be reported by the major provider of care. If the major focus is the patient's medical condition, for example, the meeting is led by a physician, nurse practitioner, or physician assistant who introduces the team to the patient and family members. Frequently, a physician, nurse practitioner, or physician assistant collaborate to discover what medical conditions a patient has, to tell the team (including differential diagnoses), and to explain how these conditions affect care (Bakerjian, 2020).

Medical orders are written with the input of the team. The physician or one of the provider team members must issue medical orders that have been agreed upon through the team process, and the physician or one of the provider team members must share team choices with the patient, family, and carers. If the main concern is nursing care, such as wound care, the nurse should take the lead in the team discussion (Bakerjian, 2020).

A virtual team can be employed if a formally established interdisciplinary team is not available or possible. A primary care physician normally leads such teams, but an advanced practice nurse or physician assistant, a care coordinator, or a case manager can form and manage them. The virtual team communicates and collaborates with team members in the community or within a health care system using information technology (e.g., handheld devices, email, video conferencing, teleconferencing) (Bakerjian, 2020).

The Geriatric Health Care Team is composed of: the gerontologist/Geriatrician, the Nurse Gerontologist, Occupational therapist, physical therapist, speech therapist, case manager, the family and other interdisciplinary team members

A *Geriatrician* is a doctor that specializes in the treatment of the elderly and the ailments that they suffer from. A multidisciplinary team is usually included in the approach, which is holistic. The geriatrician's main focus is on treating the patient's medical issues (Johns Hopkins Medicine, 2021).

A *Gerontology Nurse* is a nurse that specializes in working with senior citizens to provide specialized care and a high quality of life. Gerontology-focused advanced practice nurses work in a variety of contexts. Private practices, private houses, and nursing homes are examples of these situations (Best Master of Science in Nursing Degrees, 2015)

An *Occupational Therapist (OT)* is a health-care practitioner who helps patients achieve independence, meaningful vocations, and the functional ability to carry out their daily tasks and activities. Occupational therapists guarantee that their patient-centered interventions are effective. They've had extensive instruction in the psychological, physical, emotional, and social aspects of human behavior. OTs are also well-versed in treating the entire body using neurological principles, anatomical or physiological notions, and psychological viewpoints. Pediatrics, orthopedics, neurology, and geriatrics are among the specialties in which they practice (Regis College, n.d.).

A *Physical Therapists (PT)* is a professional that specializes in examining and treating human body diseases mostly through physical techniques. A physical therapist concentrates largely on those patients who have altered function or impairment related to the musculoskeletal, neurological, cardiovascular, and integumentary systems, whether the issue is caused by accident, disease, or other factors. A physical therapist also assesses the functioning of these systems and prescribes the best treatment to relieve pain and improve physical function (What Is a Physical Therapist, 2020)

Speech Therapist works with patients across multiple age groups to facilitate the treatment of speech and language impairments. To identify the area of issue and provide appropriate therapy or treatment, a speech therapist evaluates speech, language, cognitive-communication, and oral/feeding/swallowing skills of a client (Aged Care News, n.d.).

Case Managers are professionals that help seniors, individuals with disabilities, and their families prepare for and implement strategies that promote the best possible health, safety, independence, and quality of life. Case managers review and implement plans to meet day-to-day requirements. They also keep in touch with family members on a regular basis and develop an overall care plan to intervene in a crisis or emergency. They also put together a care team and collaborate with them to create a complete care plan for older adults (Case Management Services, n.d.).

Interdisciplinary team is made up of health care specialists from several professions who collaborate to achieve a shared goal for the patient, such as a dietician, dentist, psychologist, social worker, Neurologist, Oncologist, Surgeon, and so on (Healthcare Basics, n.d.).

Family members/Significant others are part of the health-care team because they provide psychological, emotional, physical, spiritual, and financial support to older adults (Gitlin and Wolff, 2012).

SUMMARY: As the likelihood of developing illnesses and diseases grows as one gets older, there is a greater need for older clients to receive effective and complete health care. This could be accomplished through the efforts and participation of the geriatric health care team, which is made up of professionals who specialize in different areas. Doctors, nurses, therapists, and others may make up the geriatric team, but everyone has a responsibility to play in addressing the problems and issues of the elderly.

Learning Activity: Reflect on the following questions and answer as honestly as you can.

1. What do you think will be the result if the health care team lacks collaboration?

2. Other than collaboration, what necessary factors can you identify to make the health care team work in addressing the needs of an elder client?

Case Study 1: Mr. Romero, a veteran army officer, suffered a stroke the day before yesterday. As a result of the stroke, he suffers right-sided paresthesia and slurred speech. He has trouble digesting solid foods and requires assistance when urinating. Mr. Romero requires assistance when ambulating due to his paresthesia.

Question: What members of the health-care team do you believe are required to offer Mr. Romero with holistic and complete care? Explain.

Chapter 9
RESEARCH AGENDA ON AGING

Overview

The elderly (those aged 60 and up) serve as a conduit for the transmission of generational legacies from one generation to the next. Whatever decent society we have today is a reflection of the humanism that older people have fostered during their lives. The Philippines is a country that values senior citizens as a valuable human resource. The importance of the elderly in the growth of their families and communities cannot be overstated in a culture that views the family as the basic unit of society. As a result, the Philippines recognizes the importance of putting in place policies and programs that not only ensure that the elderly have access to adequate social services and raise their standard of living, but also provide opportunities for continued and active participation in national development.

Learning Objectives:

At the end of the learning activity, you will be able to:

1. Identify current research agenda on aging
2. List some current research publications on aging
3. Extrapolate implications of current research findings on aging to the nursing practice

Subject Matter

A. National: NIH Publication-2030 Problems on Caring for Aging Baby Boomers
B. International: UN Program on Aging

C. Other Current Research on Aging

RESEARCH AGENDA ON AGING

A. NATIONAL: NIH PUBLICATION-2030 PROBLEMS ON CARING FOR AGING BABY BOOMERS

Baby Boomers

Baby Boomer is defined as "a person born during a period of time in which there is a marked rise in a population's birthrate", "usually considered to be in the years from 1946 to 1964 (Merriam-Webster Dictionary). The baby boomer generation accounts for a sizable fraction of the global population, particularly in developed countries. Baby boomers are approaching retirement age and are confronted with a number of issues, including health care (Sandeen, 2008).

In the next 10 to 15 years, the baby boomers will retire, and they will be moving the economy in the direction of health and wellness. As this group prepares for their golden years, demand for travel and leisure, gym and spa subscriptions, health supplements, anti-aging cosmetics, and retirement and vacation houses has increased in recent years. According to a study conducted by the Philippine Retirement Authority, about 778,961 baby boomers will retire globally by 2025 (Baby Boomers, Retirement and Real Estate, n.d.).

The 2030 Agenda for Sustainable Development and Older Persons

Preparing for an ageing population is critical to achieving the integrated 2030 Agenda's goals of poverty eradication, excellent health, gender equality, economic development and decent jobs, decreased disparities, and sustainable cities, as ageing cuts across all of them. While it is critical to address the exclusion and vulnerability of many older people, as well as prejudice against them, it is even more critical to go beyond considering them as a vulnerable group in the execution of the new agenda. In order to achieve really transformative, inclusive, and sustainable development outcomes, older people must be regarded as active agents of society progress (HelpAge International, n.d.).

The 2030 Program for Sustainable Development, which was just adopted, is a comprehensive development agenda that focuses on reducing inequality and reaching all demographic groups, particularly the most vulnerable. The Millennium Development Goals (MDGs) have been replaced with the Sustainable Development Goals (SDGs) (MDGs). From 2016 through 2030, this universal agenda will drive countries and international development actors in their efforts to combat extreme poverty, inequality, and climate change (HelpAge International, n.d.).

The 2030 Agenda for Sustainable Development lays out a comprehensive strategy to achieve sustainable development in a balanced manner while also ensuring that all people's human rights are respected. It emphasizes the importance of leaving no one behind and ensuring that the Sustainable Development Goals (SDGs) are realized for all parts of society, at all ages, with a special focus on the most vulnerable, such as the elderly (HelpAge International, n.d.).

Several goals of the Sustainable Development Goals address the concerns of older people, including those linked to social safety, health, decreasing disparities, and ending poverty (Goals 1, 3, 10, and 11). Nutrition, resource consumption, healthcare, accessibility, safety, and age-specific data collecting and analysis are all targets that include older people (HelpAge International, n.d.).

The 2030 Agenda places inclusion at the forefront of the agenda by repeating the phrase "... for all" in practically every goal. Several of the goals, such as Goal 3 "Ensure healthy lives and promote well-being for all at all ages" and Goal 10 "Reduce inequality within and among all countries," directly or indirectly address population ageing and older people (HelpAge International, n.d.).

The Situation of Baby Boomers (Older Persons) in the Philippines

With a population of around 80 million people, the number of elderly people has constantly increased, owing to advances in health care and, as a result, greater life expectancy. An estimated 5.2 million senior Filipinos, or roughly 6.4 percent of the population, live in the country. The senior population is expected to reach 9.5 percent of the population by 2020 (United Nations, n.d.).

Filipino families have a long history of holding older people in high regard. Regardless, their unique requirements, such as health care, housing, financial security, and other social services, must be met not only by their families and communities, but also by the entire government apparatus. As a result of the pressures of economic survival on Filipino families, they are subject to maltreatment. In 1970, for every senior person, there were around 11 working persons who could provide assistance. According to research, there will only be 6 individuals of working age to support the elderly by 2020 (United Nations, n.d.).

The aged health provides the largest challenge to the government today, among the various psychosocial issues of older people. There has been a significant mortality rate from diseases that may have been avoided. Heart disease, vascular illnesses, diabetes mellitus, chronic obstructive pulmonary diseases (COPDs), and iron deficiency anemia are all common lifestyle-related ailments. The country's public health care system has not evolved effectively to satisfy the health demands of the elderly on the responder end. The ratio of geriatricians to the elderly is currently 1:186,839. In government hospitals, there is also a noticeable paucity of geriatric wards. Because most elderly people have limited incomes, they are unable to afford private health care. Furthermore, even if health-care services are accessible, the senior population's capacity to use them is limited (United Nations, n.d.).

Globalization and modernization have had a significant impact on family life. The trend of older people assuming surrogate parental duties has emerged as a result of the flight of working-age adults to occupations abroad. They have been entrusted with the task of providing parental care for their grandkids whose parents have gone overseas to work. This puts undue demand on elderly people's physical, psychosocial, and economical capacities. On the other side, due to families' limited financial resources, the elderly's needs are prioritized over those of the younger children. This puts the elderly in a disadvantageous position (United Nations, n.d.).

National Policies and Plan of Action for Older Persons

The Philippine Constitution lays out a comprehensive policy framework for elderly people. "It is the duty of the family to care for its senior members while the state may establish social security programs for them," says Article XV,

Section 4. This demonstrates the county's commitment to preventing age discrimination and promoting active aging. Older people's goals, knowledge, and energy must be successfully directed into the national economic and social development process (United Nations, 2021).

The Philippine Plan of Action for Older Persons outlined the country's vision for older people as well as the primary actions that would be taken to implement appropriate policies, strategies, processes, and programs/projects. With a chosen focal agency, the PPAOP focused on eight primary areas of concern:

Concern	Focal Agency
1. Older Persons and the Family	Department of Social Welfare and Development (DSWD)
2. Social Position of Older Persons	Department of Interior and Local Government (DILG)
3. Social Services and Community	Coalition of Social Services for the Elderly (COSE
4. Continuing Education / Learning among Older Persons	Department of Education (DepED)
5. Older Persons and the Market	Department of Trade and Industry (DTI)
6. Health and Nutrition	Department of Health (DOH)
7. Housing, Transportation and Built Environment	Department of Transportation and Communications (DOTC)
8. Income Security, Maintenance, and Employment	Department of Finance (DOF)

*Source:*https://www.mhlw.go.jp/bunya/kokusaigyomu/asean/asean/kokusai/siryou/dl/h16_philippines2.pdf

In order to incorporate ageing into development policy, the government has achieved the enactment of both the Senior Citizen's Act (RA 7432) and the Senior Citizen's Center Act (RA 7433). (RA 7876). In addition, the Expanded Senior Citizens Act of 2003 (RA 9257) was passed, amending RA 7434. Senior Citizens are given additional advantages and rights under RA 9257. These benefits include a 20% reduction on all prices of goods and services supplied to the general public, regardless of the quantity purchased from any of the senior citizen's preferred institutions (Lucentales, n.d.).

They are also excluded from paying income taxes and have access to free medical and dental care in government facilities, as well as a 20% discount on air and sea transportation. Elderly people who want to continue their education are also given educational rights. These are in addition to the social security benefits provided to pensioners. The availability of these benefits is ensured by several government departments, but is monitored locally by each local government unit's Office of Senior Citizens Affairs (OSCA) (Lucentales, n.d.).

B. INTERNATIONAL: UN PROGRAM ON AGING

The United Nations General Assembly declared October 1 as International Day of Older Persons on December 14, 1990. Initiatives like the Vienna International Plan of Action on Ageing, which was established by the World Assembly on Ageing in 1982 and endorsed by the UN General Assembly later that year, came before it (United Nations, 2021).

The United Nations Principles for Older Persons were adopted by the General Assembly in 1991 (United Nations, 2021).

The Madrid International Plan of Action on Ageing was approved by the Second World Assembly on Ageing in 2002 to react to the potential and difficulties of population ageing in the twenty-first century and to support the development of a society for all ages (United Nations, 2021).

At all levels, the main United Nations conferences and summits, as well as special sessions of the General Assembly and review follow-up processes, have established goals, objectives, and commitments aimed at improving everyone's economic and social circumstances. These establish the context in which older people's contributions and concerns must be considered. If their provisions are implemented, older people will be able to contribute completely and profit equitably from progress (United Nations, 2021).

The International Plan of Action on Aging, 2002, has a number of fundamental themes that are linked to these aims, objectives, and commitments, including:

a) The full realization of all human rights and fundamental freedoms of all older persons;
b) The achievement of secure ageing, which involves reaffirming the goal of eradicating poverty in old age and building on the United Nations Principles for Older Persons;
c) Empowerment of older persons to fully and effectively participate in the economic, political and social lives of their societies, including through income-generating and voluntary work;
d) Provision of opportunities for individual development, self-fulfillment and well-being throughout life as well as in late life, through for example, access to lifelong learning and participation in the community while recognizing that older persons are not one homogenous group;
e) Ensuring the full enjoyment of economic, social and cultural rights, and civil and political rights of persons and the elimination of all forms of violence and discrimination against older persons;
f) Commitment to gender equality among older persons through, inter alia, elimination of gender-based discrimination;
g) Recognition of the crucial importance of families, intergenerational interdependence, solidarity and reciprocity for social development;
h) Provision of health care, support and social protection for older persons, including preventive and rehabilitative health care;
i) Facilitating partnership between all levels of government, civil society, the private sector and older persons themselves in translating the International Plan of Action into practical action;
j) Harnessing of scientific research and expertise and realizing the potential of technology to focus on, inter alia, the individual, social and health implications of ageing, in particular in developing countries;
k) Recognition of the situation of ageing indigenous persons, their unique circumstances and the need to seek means to give them an effective voice in decisions directly affecting them (United Nations, 2021).

C. **OTHER CURRENT RESEARCH ON AGING**

In a two-year study, the Institute of Medicine (IOM) brought together 87 experts from various fields related to aging and age-related research to identify the needs and opportunities for aging research in basic biomedical science, social and behavioral sciences, clinical medicine, health care delivery, and biomedical ethics. The goal of the group was to chronicle and summarize recent interesting breakthroughs in aging research in order to establish clear research objectives for the future.

The area of research must have fit into one or more of the following main categories to be considered for a significant spot on the National Research Agenda on Aging:

a) *General aging processes:* Such studies focus on theories of aging (diverse mechanisms of aging processes, including genetic and environmental components and their interaction) functioning at the molecular, cellular, organ, organ system, organism, and wider psychosocial and sociocultural levels.

b) *Important age-related disease:* This might be a disease occurring predominantly in aged populations or a disease found across the lifespan whose occurrence in old age is associated with specific alterations in its presentation, course, or sequelae (e.g., diabetes).

c) *Factors influencing age-disease interaction:* A number of lifestyle and socio-environmental factors have an important influence both on the emergence of disease in aging populations and on the mode of presentation by the older victims of disease.

d) *The functional capacity of the elderly:* The enormous importance of functional capacity as a determinant of the care needs of older persons dictates a special focus on those factors that limit the activity of elderly individuals and impair their independence (The National Academies Press, n.d.).

During its deliberations, the IOM committee identified 11 emerging and overarching themes relevant to the entire spectrum of research on aging; some of them are the following:

a. *An interdisciplinary approach to aging research:* Only an interdisciplinary group can adequately address many of the most intractable challenges in aging research, notably in the clinical, social, and behavioral arenas.

Interdisciplinary research is more expensive and difficult to design and carry out successfully than unidisciplinary research.

b. *Increasing the corpus of data based on longitudinal research:* Much of the information on aging that is now accessible is based on cross-cohort studies that compare people of different ages. Although these studies provide some insight into the impacts of aging, they are influenced by factors other than age, such as secular and cohort effects. Longitudinal studies, in which the same individuals are measured repeatedly throughout time, give a far more robust approach to gerontologic and geriatric research.

c. *Neglectful factors such as gender, race, cultural background, and ethnicity:* To understand the mechanisms behind disparities in the appearance, course, and outcomes of a number of geriatric-related illnesses, more study on aging in people of diverse racial, cultural, and ethnic groups is needed. Gender has also been proven to have a significant impact on biological, social, and behavioral elements of aging.

d. *Research into the role of genetics, social factors, and environmental variables in aging:* The impacts of aging have been exaggerated, while the modifying influences of an individual's genetic background, dietary status, exercise, personal habits, and psychosocial factors have been overlooked.

e. *The individual's psychological and sociological context:* Interdisciplinary approaches that take into account both the individual's behavior and surroundings, as well as social connections and support structures, will be critical. The requirement to explain specific age-related findings is also critical.

f. *As a study topic, ethical considerations in the care of the elderly:* Previous research agendas on aging have largely ignored ethical considerations such as health-care rationing, the provision of care to and the conduct of study on demented and irreversibly ill older people, particularly when it comes to the use of life-sustaining technologies.

g. *Research on elder populations on health promotion and disease prevention:* There has already been a revolutionary improvement in life expectancy. An increase in active life expectancy as a result (The National Academies Press, n.d.).

RESEARCH ON AGING IN THE PHILIPPINES

Aging in the Philippines is still an issue with a lot of unanswered questions (Villegas, 2014). Despite the fact that older Filipinos appear in national reports, empirical studies including older individuals appear to be rare in the Philippines. The Philippines' major universities have research institutes that investigate a variety of themes; however, the University of the Philippines Manila is now the only large university having a dedicated aging research center. The majority of study on older Filipinos tends to be focused on aging perspectives, older Filipinos' quality of life, and older persons in the labor (Badana & Andel, 2018).

SUMMARY: The world's population is increasingly aging. Many countries, including the Philippines, are increasingly preparing for the aging population. Changing demographics pose social and economic difficulties, not least for healthcare. The idea of an ageing population is frequently framed in terms of increased expectations and pressures. While adjusting will be difficult, the overall picture is not bleak if policymakers make smart changes. Individually, most individuals want a longer lifespan. Even if many of people living longer have long-term problems, they manage them well. That is, old age is not an illness. Despite living longer than any previous generation, the baby boomers are not eager to retire at 65 and attend a nursing facility. This chapter has discussed some of the difficulties facing healthcare as the world ages.

Learning Activity: Reflect on the following question and answer as honestly as you can.

Do you think there are more aging issues that need to be part of the research agenda on the developments in aging research?

Guiding Question:

Write a policy paper on senior citizen-friendly healthcare policies that can be adopted in your area, based on what was discussed in this chapter concerning the aging process, aging challenges, and aging care.

Chapter 10
TRENDS/ISSUES AND CHALLENGES ON THE CARE OF OLDER PERSONS

Overview:

Growing older has numerous difficulties. Losing their independence, physical ability deterioration, and age discrimination are only few of the difficulties people confront as they age. This growing older adult population will have an increasing need for health care and healthcare-related services, which will be felt primarily by our society as we grapple with the implications of caring for our elderly. The rising proportion of older individuals in the population need not create serious issues provided we provide suitable resources for older adults' quality of life, such as specialized healthcare facilities. Elder care, or simply eldercare, is the provision of services to meet the unique needs and requirements of older adults or senior citizens. This broad word refers to in-home care, hospice care, adult daycare, and assisted living.

Learning Objectives:

At the end of the learning activity, you will be able to:

1. Identify current trends, issues and challenges in the care of older persons
2. Differentiate home care services for older people with different health needs

Subject Matter

    A. Home Care

B. Hospice Facility
C. Drop-in/ Day Care Centers
D. Retirement Living/ Home Village

TRENDS/ISSUES AND CHALLENGES ON THE CARE OF OLDER PERSONS

A. HOME HEALTH CARE

Home healthcare enables older persons to maintain their independence as long as possible, even when they are ill or injured. It encompasses a broad range of services and frequently serves to postpone the need for long-term nursing home care (Home Health Care, n.d.).

Occupational and physical therapy, speech therapy, and skilled nursing are all examples of home health care. It may entail assisting elderly persons with daily living activities like as bathing, dressing, and eating. Additionally, it may involve assistance with cooking, cleaning, and other household tasks, as well as prescription monitoring (Home Health Care, n.d.).

It is critical to distinguish between home health care and home care services. While home health care may involve some forms of home care, it is primarily medical in nature. While home care services include household duties and cleaning, home health care typically entails assisting someone in recovering from an illness or injury. Professionals in home health care are frequently licensed practical nurses, therapists, or home health aides. The majority of them work for state-licensed home health organizations, hospitals, or public health authorities (Home Health Care, n.d.).

Types of Home Health Care Services

The spectrum of home health care options available to patients is virtually unlimited. Care may range from nursing care to specialized medical services such as laboratory workups, depending on the patient's situation. You and your doctor will decide on your care plan and any in-home services that may be necessary. Among the services available for in-home care are the following:

- *Doctor care.* A physician may come to a patient's house to diagnose and treat a disease(es). He or she may also examine the needs for home health care on a regular basis.

- *Nursing care (assistance).* The most prevalent sort of home health care is nursing care, which varies depending on the individual's needs. A registered nurse will create a care plan in cooperation with the doctor. Wound dressing, ostomy care, intravenous therapy, drug administration, monitoring the patient's overall health, pain control, and other health assistance are all examples of nursing care.

- *Occupational, physical, and/or speech therapy.* Following an illness or accident, some people may require assistance in relearning how to do daily tasks or improving their voice. A physical therapist can devise a treatment plan to assist a patient regain or strengthen muscle and joint function. An occupational therapist can assist a patient with physical, developmental, social, or emotional problems in relearning daily tasks such as eating, bathing, dressing, and other activities. A speech therapist can help a patient who has lost their capacity to communicate clearly regain it.

- *Social and medical services.* Medical social workers assist patients with a variety of services, including counseling and locating community resources to aid in their recovery. If the patient's medical condition is complex and requires the coordination of multiple services, some social workers also serve as the patient's case manager.

- *Care from home health aides.* The patient's fundamental personal needs, such as getting out of bed, walking, showering, and dressing, can be assisted by home health aides. Under the direction of a nurse, some aides have obtained additional training to assist with more specialized care.

- *Homemaker or basic assistance care.* While a patient is receiving medical treatment at home, a homemaker or someone who assists with duties or responsibilities can keep the household running smoothly by preparing meals, doing laundry, grocery shopping, and other housekeeping tasks.

- *Companionship.* Some patients who are alone at home may require the company and supervision of a companion. Some companions may also help out around the house.
- *Volunteer care.* Companionship, personal care, transportation, emotional support, and/or administrative assistance are all examples of how volunteers from community organizations can provide basic comfort to the patient.

- *Nutritional support.* Dietitians might visit a patient at home to conduct dietary assessments and provide advice to help them stick to their treatment plan.

- *Laboratory and X-ray imaging.* Certain laboratory procedures, such as blood and urine tests, can be done at the patient's own home. Furthermore, lab technicians can conduct this service at home using portable X-ray devices.

- *Pharmaceutical services.* Medical supplies and equipment might be delivered to your home. If the patient needs it, instruction in the administration of medications or the use of equipment, including intravenous therapy, can be provided.

- *Transportation.* There are companies that offer transportation to and from medical facilities for treatment or physical tests.

- *Home-delivered meals.* Many towns provide this service, known as Meals-on-Wheels, to patients at home who are unable to cook for themselves. Hot meals can be provided several times a week, depending on the individual's needs (Johns Hopkins Medicine, 2021)

B. **HOSPICE FACILITY**

Hospice care, according to the National Hospice and Palliative Care Organization, is end-of-life care for a terminal patient. Hospice care is delivered in a holistic manner, which implies that it is provided by a group of professionals. A hospice team typically includes physicians, nurse practitioners, home health providers, social workers, preachers, and family members (National Institute on Aging, 2021).

Hospice care is not intended to treat a patient who has been diagnosed with a terminal illness or a chronic condition. When a person has less than six months to live, it is important give compassionate care that satisfies varied demands. Hospice provides spiritual and emotional support, pain management, and medical therapy through the coordination of the team. In the end, hospice is designed to allow people to die with dignity and without agony. As a result, when elders choose hospice care, they forfeit their entitlement to additional treatment or remedies for their illness (National Institute on Aging, 2021).

Hospice Care vs. Palliative Care

Hospice and palliative care are commonly confused, although they are not the same sorts of senior care. This is because both types of care entail a group of people working together to support a person who is suffering from a serious illness. Palliative care, on the other hand, begins when a patient begins therapy for a disease such as cancer or kidney failure. The purpose of palliative care is to provide comfort through a holistic approach while the patient receives treatment (National Institute on Aging, 2021).

Hospice Care vs. Comfort Care

A medical doctor or nurse may use the word "comfort care" to refer to hospice care. They may refer to end-of-life care as comfort care because that is essentially what hospice is all about: offering comfort to the patient rather than curing their condition (National Institute on Aging, 2021).

When Should Hospice Care be Considered?

The decision to receive hospice care is significant because it tries to bring comfort towards the end of life with a terminal disease. Once a patient is admitted to hospice, he or she is no longer eligible for medical treatments or cures that could help them recover from their sickness or condition. Only pain management and patient comfort treatments will be given to them (National Institute on Aging, 2021).

Types of Hospice Care

a. *Hospice Care in Nursing Homes.* Hospice care can be provided in nursing homes. A nursing home, on the other hand, is not a hospice care facility. Nursing homes give seniors with a place to reside while they receive treatment or long-term care. A hospice team is established for end-of-life care when a senior is no longer responding to treatment and has been found to have less than six months to live. As a result, patients receiving hospice care might remain in a nursing home.

b. *In-Home Hospice Care.* Hospice services can be provided to older people who reside at home. The elderly individual is not required to enter a hospice facility. This is the most comfortable option for those who choose to die at home. In fact, transferring a person who is nearing the end of their life from their home to a medical institution is usually the last option. Instead, hospice nurses can collaborate with home care professionals to provide comfort to elders in their own homes.

The hospice nurse will collaborate with a team of church leaders, family members, and medical experts to offer care for the patient in their home. If the senior requires immediate medical attention or services deemed necessary for their comfort, they may be sent to a hospital. The patient may die while in the hospital, depending on his or her medical state. However, the senior's health care demands and comfort level are the sole determinants (National Institute on Aging, 2021).

Hospice Services and Benefits

Patients can choose from a variety of services provided by hospice care providers. This can entail providing care for the senior in their own home as well as medical equipment and supplies such as hospital beds and wheelchairs. In addition to daily care, hospice services may include social assistance and counseling, as well as a homemaker and home health assistant. Insurance, particularly Medicaid, may support physical therapy, speech-language pathology, and occupational therapy. These therapies, on the other hand, can only be used to provide comfort to the patient and not as a cure or treatment (National Institute on Aging, 2021).

When a senior is admitted to hospice care, a team is put together to give comfort and care. A hospice nurse and a medical doctor are part of this team, and both are available 24 hours a day, 7 days a week for questions or assistance. There will also be someone who is always with the patient. A home care nurse, for example, might be with the patient from 8 a.m. to 8 p.m., and then a family member would spend the night with the patient. Residents of a nursing home or hospice facility will be constantly monitored by the organization's employees (National Institute on Aging, 2021).

Because hospice care focuses on end-of-life care, it usually focuses on pain management for the patient. The hospice team will also do everything possible to ensure the person's comfort. Let's say the senior is having trouble with their faith or is worried about what will happen when they die. In that situation, they will be visited by a clergy leader or a member of their own church who will answer their questions and provide spiritual assistance (National Institute on Aging, 2021).

If a patient wishes to see all of their family members before dying, the team will do all possible to accommodate them. They may, for example, give video conferencing or telephone conversations to allow communications with people who live out of town or who are unable to visit the senior. The hospice team is dedicated to satisfying any and all of the patient's needs in order to ensure that they are comfortable and can die with dignity (National Institute on Aging, 2021).

C. DROP-IN/DAYCARE CENTERS

Adult daycare is a structured program of activities for older persons who require supervised care throughout the day or who are solitary and lonely. It is provided in a professional setting. Adult daycare centers allow seniors to mingle and participate in organized activities in a group setting while also obtaining necessary medical care. At the same time, they allow family caregivers a break from caring for their loved ones while ensuring that they are safe (HelpGuide.org., 2020).

The level of care provided varies depending on the facility. While one sort of center concentrates mostly on social and recreational services, with a few health-related and personal care services thrown in for good measure, another will offer a more comprehensive range of medical and therapeutic services. Physical, occupational, or speech therapy, for example, or medical treatments provided by a registered nurse or other health professional, are examples of these services. Finally, a third type of facility will provide specialized care for persons who have a medical condition, such as dementia or a handicap. Adult day care centers are typically open during the day from Monday to Friday, while some services may be accessible on weekends or evenings (HelpGuide.org., 2020).

Goals of Drop-in/ Day Care Centers

Whatever services are offered, the goal is basically twofold:

a. To allow older persons to go out of the house and gain both mental and social stimulation, as well as the ongoing care they require.
b. To offer caregivers a much-needed respite so they can work, take care of personal matters, or simply rest and relax (HelpGuide.org., 2020).

Services provided by adult day care centers

The goals of a well-run adult day care facility will be to enrich the lives of participants, build on their skills and abilities, and provide plenty of social interaction. The features of each institution vary, but services may include:

a. *Social activities.* Planned activities are usually adapted to the abilities and health circumstances of the participants. Arts and crafts, musical entertainment and sing-alongs, mental stimulation activities like bingo, stretching or other light exercise, discussion groups (for books, films, or current events, for example), holiday and birthday celebrations, and local outings are all possibilities.

b. *Nutrition.* Seniors in day care centers receive nutritious meals, including those that cater to particular diets, as well as snacks.

c. *Personal care (hygiene).* Grooming, bathroom hygiene, walking, and feeding are all activities that center personnel can assist with.

d. *Health-care services.* Medication dispensing, blood pressure monitoring, hearing checks, and vision screening are just some of the services available, as are symptom management and more intense medical or therapy services.

e. *Transportation.* Some adult day care centers offer transportation to and from the facility, as well as to any area outings.

f. *Caregivers' services.* Some centers may offer counseling, caregiver support groups, assistance with care planning, and caregiver education. A well-run adult day care center's goals will focus on enriching participants' lives, building upon their skills and strengths, and providing lots of social interaction (HelpGuide.org., 2020).

When to consider adult day care

When an older person needs help, he or she may wish to seek adult day care.

   a. Can no longer plan their own daily activities
   b. Feels lonely and seeks companionship
   c. Cannot be left alone at home.
   d. Lives with a partner who works outside the home or is regularly away for other reasons.

Adult day care centers are a good fit for older people who:

   a. Can benefit from the camaraderie and practical help provided by a day care center.
   b. Despite the fact that they may be physically or mentally impaired, they do not require round-the-clock monitoring.
   c. Are suffering from Alzheimer's disease in its early stages.
   d. Are mobile, with the use of a cane, walker, or wheelchair if necessary.
   e. Are there any continents? (in most cases).

D. RETIREMENT LIVING/ HOME VILLAGE

A retirement home, also known as an old people's home or an old age home, is a multi-residence living facility for the elderly. The term "retirement house" can also apply to a nursing home. Each person or couple in the house usually has their own apartment-style room or suite of rooms (SeniorLiving.org., 2019).

Each person or couple in a retirement home lives in an apartment-style room or suite of rooms, which often includes a living space, bedrooms, bathrooms, and a small kitchen or kitchenette. There may also be studio flats with a combined living space, bedroom, and kitchenette (SeniorLiving.org., 2019).

Communal food, some sort of healthcare, organized recreational activities, spa services, hairdresser services, transportation, and other amenities and services are provided within each privately-owned facility. The amenities and services available vary by area. In a nutshell, a retirement home is a facility where senior citizens can live and get care and support (SeniorLiving.org., 2019).

Types of Retirement Homes:

Each senior has his or her own set of requirements, wants, and desires. Various types of retirement homes provide a variety of options for meeting those needs.

a. *Religious or faith-based retirement homes.* Many people, especially as they get older, find it helpful to have the support of others who share their beliefs. For those whose faith is important in their lives, a faith-based or religious-based retirement home may be a better fit.

   Faith-based communities provide people with a built-in support structure. They call you when you're sick to see if you need anything. Someone is willing to help you run errands. They are there to provide you with the assistance you require, regardless of the situation.

b. *Masonic Retirement Residences.* Although many Retirement Homes were founded to assist persons linked with Freemasonry, many have now opened their doors to non-Masonic members, however this varies by region. Non-Masons (the general public) are often given lower priority than Masons and their families (waiting lines can be long), and they are not eligible for the discounts offered to Masons and their families.

c. *Retirement Homes for Veterans.* Although many veterans choose to live among the general public, some prefer to live in communities dedicated solely to veterans. The capacity of a veteran to live in a veteran retirement home is determined by eligibility criteria. Age, military rank and status, criminal history, and physical and mental health at the time of entry are all considered.

d. *Luxury Retirement Homes.* There are numerous levels and types of luxury in Luxury Retirement Homes. Residents of luxury retirement homes have a luxurious place to live and a more than comfortable place to return to after chasing all of your other retirement aspirations (SeniorLiving.org., 2019).

SUMMARY: Changes in living settings are anticipated to occur as the prevalence of chronic and acute illnesses among older persons increases, as does the resulting deterioration in functional status and the multiple losses suffered by older adults. Many seniors continue to live independently at home or with the assistance of a caregiver. Changing the environment is frequently required for financial reasons. In some circumstances, older persons may need to relocate in order to access health treatment or a more functioning, supportive environment. For older persons, transitioning from one environment to another can be stressful, unpleasant, and result in negative health and emotional results. Older individuals can be found in a variety of settings.

Learning Activity: Reflect on the following questions and answer as honestly as you can.

1. Have you ever cared for an older adult? If so, what was that experience like? How do you feel about caring for older adults in your nursing practice?
2. What do you think about nurses who work in nursing homes? Have you ever considered a career in gerontology? What are the positives you can see about developing expertise in this field of nursing?
3. Which of the settings for gerontologic nursing practice appeal to you most at this time that might influence you in your professional career in the future? Is there any one setting that you can see yourself working in more than another? Do you think this will change as you progress in your career?

Case Study 1: The Reyes family is a close-knit group of five, with Papa B., their grandfather, living with them in their house since he was widowed ten years ago. Papa B. is 88 years old and has just been diagnosed with early-stage Alzheimer's disease. Papa B. is becoming increasingly difficult to supervise, and the family believes it is no longer safe for him to be alone at home. Both parents work during the day, and the three children attend high school during the day. The family wants to keep Papa B. at home, but they do not know what resources are available in the community to assist them.

Questions:

1. What services might the Reyes family use to help them keep Papa B. at home? Do these services seem feasible at this time?
2. As Papa B.'s condition worsens with the progression of Alzheimer's disease, what other services discussed in this chapter might be necessary at various points in time?
3. What assessments would a nurse need to make in order to determine the best placement for Papa B.? Given the history of this family, what recommendations for the future might be made? Which interdisciplinary team member could provide additional information to the nurse and the family about community services?

Case Study 2: Mrs. Hobson, who has lived in her home for the past 60 years, is 89 years old. Her husband died 25 years ago, and she now relies on her two sons and daughter to help her with groceries and transportation to medical appointments. She is self-sufficient in all aspects of her daily life. She lives in an inner-city neighborhood that has significantly degraded throughout her stay there. Mrs. Hobson's house was broken into last night. Mrs. Hobson surprised the burglar, and the crowbar used to shatter the window and enter the house struck her in the head. She was taken to the hospital's emergency room and then sent home.

Questions:
1. What is Mrs. Hobson's biggest challenge now that she is living alone?
2. What other home options may Mrs. Hobson think about?
3. What consequences may Mrs. Hobson encounter if she moved to a more supportive environment?
4. What interventions could be undertaken to make Mrs. Hobson safer and enable her to function at the highest level of independence if she were to remain in her own home

Chapter 11
ADVOCACY PROGRAMS RELEVANT TO THE CARE OF OLDER PERSONS

Overview

The older adults are considered to be one of the most vulnerable groups. As a result, individuals experience difficulties in their daily life. Elder abuse in nursing homes, a lack of access to medication and healthcare, and transportation issues are just a few of the hurdles that some older people experience. Advocates assist the elderly by focusing on critical issues and raising public awareness. The ways in which nurses can advocate for their elderly patients as well as the mental health services for the elderly are discussed in this chapter.

Learning Objectives:

At the end of the learning activity, you will be able to:

1. Identify advocacy programs relevant to the care of older persons
2. List the DOH health programs for the senior citizens of the country

Subject Matter

A. Support Services And Advocacy For Older People
B. Mental Health Programs

ADVOCACY PROGRAMS RELEVANT TO THE CARE OF OLDER PERSONS

A. <u>SUPPORT SERVICES AND ADVOCACY FOR OLDER PEOPLE</u>

An *advocate* is a neutral third party who can assist older people in understanding and asserting their rights in the aged care system. This involves ensuring that the elderly person has a say in important decisions, giving options for meeting their aged care needs, and assisting them in resolving complaints and issues (New Homepage, 2021).

Advocacy services

Advocacy services protect the rights of everyone who is receiving or requesting aged care services, and they enable older persons to make informed decisions about their care (New Homepage, 2021).

What can an advocate do?

An aged care advocate can assist older persons with things like:

a. Interacting with the aged care system
b. Transitioning between aged care services
c. Knowing and understanding rights of older persons
d. Making decisions about the care received by older persons
e. Options for having the older person's aged care needs better met
f. Resolving concerns or complaints with the older person's aged care provider about the services they receive.
g. Speaking with the service provider of the older persons
h. Increasing the older person's skills and knowledge to advocate for themselves (New Homepage, 2021).

Who can access advocacy services?

Advocacy services are available to anyone receiving or requesting government-funded aged care services, including family and representatives. This includes those who:

a. they live in an aged care facility;
b. they receive aged care services in their own home;
c. they receive transition care; and
d. they assist someone who is receiving aged care services (New Homepage, 2021).

HOW TO BECOME AN ADVOCATE FOR OLDER PERSONS

Method 1: Assisting with Day-to-Day Activities

a) *Work in a nursing home as a volunteer.* By conversing with and spending time with the elderly, you will gain a better understanding of their everyday struggles and worries. Concerns about healthcare, common health difficulties like dementia, unmet nutritional needs, social isolation, and a persistent need for physical or recreational activities are all things you might notice.

b) *Volunteer to assist elderly people who are self-sufficient.* While many seniors choose to live in a nursing home, others want to live at home and be self-sufficient. Working with a local organization or individually contacting specific elders you know can let you volunteer to assist them with domestic responsibilities.

c) *Acquire a basic understanding of medical procedures.* Healthcare is an important aspect of senior care, and understanding about healthcare practices and policies can help you improve the lives of the seniors with whom you live or work. Learn more about senior care by being certified in senior first aid, CPR, and AED, or by attending healthcare conferences.

d) *Assist elderly in getting online.* One of the primary problems that seniors experience on a daily basis is that they are unable to discover or access certain services that they require due to a lack of computer literacy. Assist seniors in your community in getting Internet access and learning basic computer skills (WikiHow, 2021).

Method No. 2: Raising Community Awareness

a. *Organize community forums.* Your neighborhood community center could be a nice gathering spot for local individuals to learn about the problems that older adults face. Many libraries also have conference rooms that can be used for these kind of events.

b. *Start a blog.* Create material tailored to the requirements of the elderly using an online blogging platform. Seniors who are hesitant to share their concerns in person may be willing to do so anonymously online.

c. *Join a neighborhood group.* Join a group dedicated to making the lives of the elderly better. Typically, such groups disseminate information and articles regarding legislative issues that influence the life of senior citizens. They may also work directly with older persons to address topics that are important to them (WikiHow, 2021).

Method 3: Working Politically

a. *Work for a non-profit advocacy group.* Volunteering with or working for an organization that fosters intergenerational contact and engages in legislative lobbying is one of the finest methods to advocate for the elderly. A good location to start looking for groups and services to join is the National Council on Aging.

b. *Send a letter to legislators.* Elder financial exploitation, insufficient healthcare, neglect and senior abuse, and a lack of transportation services are all essential issues to bring to legislators' notice. Make a phone call or send a letter to your local and state lawmakers to let them know that the voting public wants more attention paid to child care.

c. *Attend local gatherings as a lobbyist.* At local political events, nonviolent protests and demonstrations are used to advocate. Collaborate with national advocacy organizations to obtain resources and establish a strategy. Then collect people to take part in your demonstration (WikiHow, 2021).

Method 4: Obtaining Employment as a Senior Advocate

a. *Decide on a care area.* You can advocate for the elderly in a variety of ways as a professional. People work as patient advocates, caretakers, or coordinators to help older people join in medical or government benefit programs.

b. *Get your credentials together.* Once you've decided on a career path, enroll in the courses or programs required to advance in your chosen field. Check with your local colleges, junior colleges, and community centers to see if they offer programs in your chosen field.

c. *Make an offer of your services.* Look for work in older communities that are underserved in your area. Check with local hospitals or nursing homes to see if your services are required, or consider working as a freelancer (WikiHow, 2021).

B. MENTAL HEALTH PROGRAMS

The global population is increasingly aging, and older individuals suffer unique physical and mental health concerns that must be addressed. Over 20% of adults aged 60 and over suffer from a mental or neurological disorder (excluding headache disorders), and mental and neurological disorders account for 6.6 percent of all disability among people aged 60 and up (Mental Health of Older Adults, 2017).

Dementia and depression, which afflict about 5% and 7% of the world's senior population, respectively, are the most frequent mental and neurological problems in this age group. Anxiety disorders impact 3.8 percent of the elderly population, substance abuse affects over 1%, and about a quarter of self-harm deaths occur in those aged 60 and up. Substance addiction issues in the elderly are frequently neglected or misdiagnosed (Mental Health of Older Adults, 2017).

Mental health issues are under-diagnosed by health-care professionals and elderly people themselves, and the stigma associated with these illnesses makes people hesitant to seek help (Mental Health of Older Adults, 2017).

Risk factors for mental health problems among older adults

Older adults may face stressors that affect everyone, as well as stressors that are especially common in later life, such as a severe continual loss of capabilities and functional capacity. Older folks, for example, may suffer from diminished mobility, chronic pain, frailty, or other health issues that necessitate long-term care. Furthermore, situations such as bereavement or a reduction in socioeconomic position with retirement are more likely to occur in older persons. All of these pressures might cause isolation, loneliness, or psychological anguish in seniors, necessitating long-term care (Mental Health of Older Adults, 2017).

Elder abuse can include physical, verbal, psychological, financial, and sexual abuse, as well as abandonment, neglect, and major loss of dignity and respect. Elder abuse can result in not only physical injuries, but also serious and potentially long-term psychological effects such as depression and anxiety (Mental Health of Older Adults, 2017).

Health promotion

Promoting Active and Healthy Aging can help improve the mental health of older people. For older individuals, mental health-specific health promotion entails developing living conditions and settings that promote wellbeing and enable them to live a healthy lifestyle. Promoting mental health is largely dependent on efforts that guarantee that older persons have the resources they require, such as (Mental Health of Older Adults, 2017):

a. Providing security and freedom;
b. Adequate housing through supportive housing policy;
c. Social support for older people and their caregivers;
d. Health and social programs targeted at vulnerable groups such as those who live alone and rural populations or who suffer from a chronic or relapsing mental or physical illness;
e. Programs to prevent and deal with elder abuse; and
f. Community development programs.

Mental health care in the community

Promoting older people's health, avoiding sickness, and managing chronic illnesses all require good general health and social care. As a result, it is critical that all health care personnel have training in dealing with age-related illnesses and disorders. Primary mental health care for older individuals at the community level is critical. Focusing on the long-term care of older persons with mental illnesses, as well as providing caregivers with education, training, and support, is also critical (Mental Health of Older Adults, 2017).

WHO works with governments to strengthen and promote mental health in older individuals, as well as to include effective solutions into policies and plans. The Global strategy and action plan on ageing and health were agreed by the World Health Assembly in 2016. One of the goals of this global plan is to connect health-care systems with the requirements of older people, both mentally and physically. Orienting health systems around intrinsic capacity and functional ability, developing and ensuring affordable access to quality older person-centered and integrated clinical care, and ensuring a sustainable and appropriately trained, deployed, and managed health work force are just a few of the key actions (Mental Health of Older Adults, 2017).

It is a commitment by all WHO Member States to take concrete initiatives to promote mental well-being, prevent mental disorders, provide care, facilitate recovery, and promote human rights for people with mental disorders, including older individuals. It has four main goals.

1. Strengthen effective leadership and governance for mental health;
2. Provide comprehensive, integrated and responsive mental health and social care services in community-based settings;
3. Implement strategies for promotion and prevention in mental health; and
4. Strengthen information systems, evidence and research for mental health (Mental Health of Older Adults, 2017).

SUMMARY: The advocacy for older people was explored in this chapter. Advocates for the elderly look into problems that older people face and work to improve their living situations. Elder abuse in nursing homes, a lack of access to medication and healthcare, and transportation issues are just a few of the hurdles that some older people experience. Advocates assist the elderly by focusing on critical issues and raising public awareness. A healthcare provider can become a senior advocate by assisting them where they live, distributing knowledge and raising interest in their community, and advocating for new legislation that protect the elderly. This chapter also covered the common mental health issues that affect the elderly, as well as the risk factors that contribute to them. Finally, programs aimed at improving the mental health of older persons were investigated.

Learning Activity: Reflect on the following questions and answer as honestly as you can.

1. Observe your environment. Do you think or feel there is age-related discrimination happening around you?
2. How about in the news? Are there reports of age-related discrimination?
3. Are you knowledgeable about your local senior-citizen party-list and what are they doing? What advocacies do they lobby for?
4. Do you think or feel there is a stigma against persons with mental health concerns or illnesses?
5. Do you know of any local NGO, which advocates for mental health awareness and issues? Do they include senior citizens as among those they lobby for? How do they lobby for their advocacy?

Chapter 12
GRANDPARENTS AS TREASURE CHEST OF VALUABLE HISTORY, VALUES, TRADITIONS AND WISDOMS

Overview

The role of grandparents in our lives was the emphasis of this chapter. It includes a discussion of how grandparents may provide their grandkids with a treasure trove of significant history, values, customs, and wisdom.

Learning Objectives:

At the end of the learning activity, you will be able to:

1. Appreciate the value, wisdom and contributions of older people.

Subject Matter

"My Lolo and Lola: Our Heritage Heroes"
The Importance of Grandparents

GRANDPARENTS AS TREASURE CHEST OF VALUABLE HISTORY, VALUES, TRADITIONS AND WISDOMS

THE IMPORTANCE OF GRANDPARENTS

According to Dr. Karl Pillemer, the link between grandparents and their grandchildren is second only to the relationship between parent and child in terms of emotional relevance. When grandparents are involved in their children's life, they benefit. Grandparents, on the other hand, reap the benefits of their relationship with their grandkids (Pillemer, 2013).

10 reasons grandparents matter more than ever:

1. Grandparents make an impact in the lives of their grandkids. Grandparents that are actively involved in their grandchildren's lives can make a significant influence in their lives. More than half of grandparents see their grandkids at least once a week, and 92% of grandparents admit to changing a grandchild's diaper. This work and effort pay off in the form of healthier and happy grandchildren.

2. *Grandparents are present in greater numbers among children.* The number of grandparents has increased in tandem with the increase in life expectancy. In 1900, only around half of American teenagers had at least two living grandparents; by 1976, that number had risen to 90%.

3. *Intergenerational households are on the rise.* Households with many generations are becoming more common. Intergenerational homes are becoming more common across the country. According to the most recent U.S. Census data, 7.5 million children lived with at least one grandmother, accounting for more than 10% of the population under the age of 18.

4. *Many children are raised by their grandparents.* According to the same census data, 2.7 million grandparents provide for their grandchildren's basic necessities (are primary caregivers). Even more look after their grandchildren on a regular basis but do not serve as primary caregivers.

5. *Grandparents have spending power.* Grandparents are a financial force to be reckoned with. They control an incredible 75% of the wealth in the United States. A significant portion of that spending power is allocated to grandkids.

6. *Grandparents Give Back to the Community.* In general, elder generations are recognized for being giving with their time and money, and grandparents are no exception. According to an American Grandparents Association (AGA) poll, grandparents give 45 percent of cash donations to NGOs and 28 percent volunteer on a regular basis. Furthermore, 15% of grandparents have volunteered to help at shelters for homeless adults.

7. *Grandparents can use a computer.* Unlike the stereotype of the doddering senior who gets lost and confused in front of anything electric or with buttons, grandparents have largely embraced the digital age's trappings.

8. *Grandparents Love their Role.* According to an AGA survey, "being a grandparent is the single most significant and satisfying thing in their life for 72 percent of grandparents."

9. *Grandparents have valuable experience.* Grandparents use their previous parenting expertise to interact with their grandchildren.

10. *Today's Grandparents are Active and Involved.* Grandparents today do not simply sit in rocking chairs with blankets on their laps; they are active. According to reports, 43% of grandparents exercise or participate in sports, while 18% dance.
    SOURCE: (*10 Reasons Grandparents Matter More than Ever,* 2021)
    https://www.aplaceformom.com/caregiverresources/articles/grandparents-matter-more-than-ever

Grandparents fill a unique role in their grandchildren's lives. According to studies, children regard grandparents as quite significant and place a high importance on their interactions with them. Furthermore, the majority of grandparents like their role.

Some of the reasons why grandparents are significant have also been mentioned:

a. *Source of morals and values.* Parents instill excellent habits and beliefs in their children, but grandparents' instructions are far more profound. Grandparents can pass on the knowledge they've gained through the years.

b. *Source of knowledge and wisdom.* Grandparents' wisdom comes from a combination of experience and age. They can teach others through stories, morality, counsel, or conversation.

c. *They play an essential role in the household.* Grandparents are really valuable. They're the parents' parents, after all! They form a special link with their grandkids by taking an active role in their upbringing.

d. *They are the most effective carers (second to the parents).* Grandparents are the ideal guardians for your children since they love them unconditionally. You won't have to worry about your children's safety if they're with their grandparents. Grandparents' love and affection for your children is incomparable to that which other relatives and close friends may feel for them.

e. *They are a link to our ancestors.* Grandparents are a vital link between us and our families, as well as the community to which we all belong. Grandparents are the best source of information about our ancestors, family memories, and new information about our parents for our children.

f. *Grandparents truly impact their grandchildren's lives.* Grandparents have a significant impact on their grandchildren's life. According to studies, up to 9 out of 10 adult grandchildren believe their grandparents had an influence on their opinions and values. The relationship that a youngster has with a grandparent shapes his or her perception of what constitutes a healthy, normal relationship. Children can learn what a true, happy connection looks like through regular contact, a sense of emotional intimacy, and constant support.

g. *Grandparents can greatly reduce household stress.* "An emotionally close relationship between grandparent and grandchild is associated with fewer symptoms of depression for both generations" according to a 2014 study at Boston College.

h. *Grandparents have a great amount of experience.* Grandparents are a valuable resource since they have a wealth of personal stories and experiences to share. Children frequently pay attention to grandparents even when they are not paying attention to their parents or other people. Grandparents can also connect a youngster to his or her cultural heritage and family history. Through their relationship with their grandparents, children gain a better understanding of who they are and where they came from.

i. *Grandparents provide a sense of security.* Having an extra layer of support, especially during difficult times, can make a significant impact in a child's life. Close grandparent-grandchild relationships during the adolescent years have been linked to fewer behavioral and emotional problems, as well as fewer social challenges with peers, according to studies. When youngsters need someone to talk to, grandparents provide an extra ear, because it is sometimes easier for children to open up and share their troubles and issues with their grandparents.

j. *Grandparents offer an affordable childcare option.* With both parents working outside the home in many families, grandparents play an increasingly important role in parenting today's children. According to the 2010 Census, approximately 2.7 million grandparents provide for a grandchild's basic requirements, while even more look after their grandkids on a daily basis. Having a grandmother function as an occasional babysitter or a hired childcare provider, if they are willing and able, gives many parents great peace of mind knowing that their children are in capable and caring hands.

SUMMARY: When it comes to their grandkids, grandparents wear many hats: babysitters, nurses, carers, playmates, friends, and even replacement parents and teachers are just a few. They have a unique position of trust that allows them to assist nurture and mold the lives of their grandkids. Spending time with their grandchildren is one of the most important things grandparents do for their grandchildren. Children gain crucial lessons from their grandparents that they will remember for the rest of their lives. While grandparents like showering their grandkids with gifts and treats, the greatest gift they can give is their time, which provides a perfect opportunity to pass on basic values, beliefs, and abilities.

Learning Activity: Reflect on the following questions and answer as honestly as you can.

1. What do your grandparents mean to you?
2. Were your grandparents formative in your growing years?
3. What pieces of wisdom did you learn from your grandparents that were crucial in your life?
4. How do you relate to your grandparents?
5. What do you believe grandparents and grandchildren can learn from each other?

Guiding Question:

The students shall interview their grandparents or eldest closest living relative of each gender. Through questions, they are expected to create and write a complete biography of their elders. It can be about anything, a unique experience or their whole life. What is important is the student captures the feelings and thoughts of their elders and reflects them in the biography they will submit.

Chapter 13
TELEHEALTH/TELEMEDICINE AND OLDER PERSONS

Overview

In the Philippines, where more than 20% of the population lives in poverty, inequity in health care delivery is a serious issue. Six out of ten Filipinos died without seeking medical assistance in 2010, according to reports. They remain physically isolated and poor places with significantly limited health-care access. Across the country, there is a low doctor-to-patient ratio. With these realities in mind, the National Telehealth Center, part of the National Institutes of Health, developed the practice of Telehealth and Telemedicine at the University of the Philippines, Manila. This chapter will discuss the benefits and drawbacks of telehealth and telemedicine, as well as the facilitators and hurdles to its usability among older persons.

Learning Objectives:

At the end of the learning activity, you will be able to:

1. Describe tele health consultation
2. Identify the advantages and disadvantages of tele health consultation for older persons

Subject Matter

      A. Telehealth and Telemedicine Defined
      B. Uses of Telemedicine
      C. Telehealth and Telemedicine in the Philippines

D. Facilitators of Telehealth Usability among Older Adults
   E. Barriers to Telehealth Usability among Older Adults

TELEHEALTH/TELEMEDICINE AND OLDER PERSONS

TELEHEALTH AND TELEMEDICINE DEFINED

The terms *telehealth* and *telemedicine* are frequently used interchangeably. The World Medical Association defines *telemedicine* as "the practice of medicine over a distance, in which interventions, diagnostic and treatment decisions, and recommendations are based on data, documents, and other information conveyed via telecommunication systems" (Cranford, 2021).

Telehealth, on the other hand, is a broader phrase that encompasses more than only curative medicine. It is taken to signify the incorporation of telecommunication networks into the practice of health protection and promotion (Cranford, 2021).

USES OF TELEMEDICINE

Telemedicine uses information and communication technology (ICT) to allow a physician, usually a general practitioner in a remote community, to consult with specialists in the Philippine General Hospital, known as domain experts (Patdu &Tenorio, 2016).

General practitioners, such as the DOH Doctor to the Barrios or the Municipal Health Officer in a rural or disadvantaged community, are able to consult with specialists at the Philippine General Hospital via SMS (short messaging system for cellular phones) or electronic mail (Patdu &Tenorio, 2016).

Radiographs and other diagnostics are sent via the internet and interpreted by specialists in other parts of the world. Telemedicine services improve access to healthcare for disadvantaged communities in geographically isolated and disadvantaged areas where physical access to health facilities may be a problem or where there is a shortage of qualified practitioners to attend to patients (Patdu &Tenorio, 2016).

Telehealth and Telemedicine in the Philippines

To improve access to health services during the Enhanced Community Quarantine, the Department of Health (DOH) and the National Privacy Commission (NPC) have developed a framework for telemedicine services (Patdu &Tenorio, 2016).

Medical consultations over the phone, chat, SMS, and other audio and visual-conferencing platforms are considered telemedicine services in the country, according to the DOH-NPC Joint Memorandum Circular. These consultations allow healthcare providers to generate electronic case reports and prescriptions (Patdu &Tenorio, 2016).

How Telehealth Can Improve Access to Elderly Care

Patients can consult with their healthcare professional remotely utilizing a telemedicine program that includes live video, audio, and instant messaging. This eliminates the need for face-to-face visits and consultations, making it easier for at-home caregivers to meet their loved ones' needs (Cranford, 2021).

Many of these at-home caregivers will have their own responsibilities, such as raising children or working. They would not have to spend as much time transporting their loved one to and from the doctor's office if they could consult with their loved one's doctor from the comfort of their own home. These can quickly provide valuable insight and knowledge to at-home healthcare providers (Cranford, 2021).

Telehealth can help families and elderly patients in the following ways:

a. Reduce the burden and cost of certain travel expenses
b. Reduce the number of unnecessary hospital visits
c. Reduce the stress put on at-home caregivers
d. Improve overall patient satisfaction

Using Telehealth to Care for the Elderly

Telehealth can help at-home caregivers better manage and treat a variety of conditions and diseases that commonly affect the elderly. While in-person visits will still be necessary in many of these circumstances, telehealth makes it easier for family caregivers to care for their loved ones by providing direct access to healthcare specialists. They can always consult with a licensed physician or specialist via telemedicine video conferencing software if they have a question regarding caring for their loved one.

Telehealth can be used to care for and manage the following conditions and diseases (Cranford, 2021)**:**

Palliative Care: Telehealth allows at-home caregivers to report on their loved one's condition as their health deteriorates while obtaining crucial comments and recommendations from healthcare professionals.

Transitional Care for Heart Failure: Following an episode of heart failure, at-home caregivers can use telehealth to stay on top of their loved one's treatment plan, which includes dispensing medications, food, physical activity, and stress management.

Chronic Disease Management: At-home caregivers can use telehealth to report on their loved one's status, offering healthcare providers insight into how their disease is progressing over time. Telehealth allows caregivers to keep track of prescriptions, food information, and mental and physical changes.

Primary Care for Frail Individuals: Patients who have difficulty moving or leaving the house can speak with healthcare specialists via telehealth about a number of basic healthcare issues and concerns, such as joint pain, muscle stiffness, medications, and accident management and prevention.

There are numerous methods for elderly people and family carers to benefit from telemedicine. Digital healthcare services eliminate the need for in-person appointments, cut healthcare costs, reduce costly emergency department visits, and improve patient satisfaction. More families will need to rely on these services to care for their elderly loved ones as more patients approach retirement age.

Facilitators of Telehealth Usability among Older Adults

Several variables contribute to older individuals' adoption of telehealth, including (Cranford, 2021):

   a. Devices that use fewer buttons
   b. Automatic transmission of information
   c. Utilizing low-tech platforms (i.e., telephone, tv)
   d. Devices that generate reminders or alerts
   e. Providing both visual and audio guidance
   f. User-friendly images appropriate for the elderly

Barriers to Telehealth Usability among Older Adults

A variety of roadblocks to telehealth technology adoption have been identified (Cranford, 2021):

   a. Font size, unusual characters (difficult to read)
   b. Bland graphics and poor color contrast
   c. Using devices with widgets (older patients lack poor fine motor eye-hand coordination)
   d. Use of a computer mouse (difficult to use with arthritic hands)
   e. Unskilled on the use of a smartphone or a computer
   f. Multiple screen transitions to complete a task
   g. Menu bars that contain several layers
   h. Inappropriate size of a smartphone (too big or too small; frail patients who have diminished grip strength may have problems handling the device).

Telehealth may also constitute a cultural shift for older persons who are not used to using technology, which must be considered when implementing telehealth. Finally, delays in answers, a lack of feedback, and technical issues can all cause patients to become frustrated and lose motivation to continue self-care monitoring activities.

SUMMARY: As they manage a variety of ailments and diseases, elderly folks may have complex healthcare needs. However, many older individuals, particularly those who live in rural areas, find it difficult to obtain healthcare. This chapter discussed the various ways elderly patients and family carers might benefit from telehealth. Digital healthcare services eliminate the need for in-person appointments, cut healthcare costs, reduce costly emergency department visits, and improve patient satisfaction. More families will need to rely on these services to care for their elderly loved ones as more patients approach retirement age.

> **Learning Activity:** Reflect on the following questions and answer as honestly as you can.
>
> 1. What are the possible barriers and challenges elderly people may face in handling telecommunication and technology?
> 2. How would you propose or help them overcome those barriers?
> 3. Do you believe it is more advantageous to use Telehealth than traditional modes?
> 4. What do you believe is the future of geriatric care in the context of rapidly emerging technologies?

Guiding Question:

Students are encouraged to work in pairs to select an older adult or geriatric to undertake a case study on. They will next mimic a telehealth conference (by phone, zoom, Facebook Messenger, or any other means of communication) in which one party will play the role of an older adult patient and the other will play the role of a nurse aiding the patient with their treatment. They will submit a recorded output (either video or audio; the important thing is that both students are heard) and a written output of the case study in which they will list the potential challenges that an older adult might face with telehealth and how they overcame those challenges, as well as why they chose the telehealth channel that they did.

Chapter 14
ENTREPRENEURIAL OPPORTUNITIES

Overview:

Many countries, including the Philippines, are coping with the problem of an aging population. Chronic illnesses, disability, and dependency are all difficulties that elderly people encounter. Some relatives are unable to provide enough care for an aging relative. Alternative techniques to caring for the aged in society include home health care companies and contracting nurse entrepreneurs. The possibilities open to nurses who desire to start their own business are discussed in this chapter.

Learning Objectives:

At the end of the learning activity, you will be able to:

1. State the potential career opportunities in catering the needs of older adult clients
2. Determine the demand of health services by older people

Subject Matter

A. Home health Agencies
B. Entrepreneurship in Nursing

ENTREPRENEURIAL OPPORTUNITIES

For many countries around the world, including the Philippines, the aging society has recently surfaced as the most pressing worry. Over the previous decade, the Philippines' senior population has been significantly growing. The elderly dependent population (aged 65 and older) accounts for 3.83 percent of the population, according to the most recent NSCB data; by 2025, the elderly will account for 10.25 percent of the population. The ramifications for Philippine growth, particularly in terms of social welfare, are tremendous. The elderly's quality of life is a significant priority here, which means that in addition to satisfying their basic survival needs of food and health, an enabling environment should be provided (HelpageAsia, 2021).

It is also worth mentioning that, rather than the government, Filipino families bear the brunt of the responsibility of caring for the elderly. The majority of individuals, especially those from marginalized groups, rely on their children, grandchildren, or other family as they get older. However, even this traditional backing is eroding in these changing times. Factors such as the family's economic and social instability increase the deterioration (HelpageAsia, 2021).

Due to the limited scope of public geriatric care and the rising cost of living, Filipino families are also under pressure to provide a good quality of life for their elderly members. Furthermore, even moderate to wealthy households are unable to effectively care for their elderly members due to a variety of challenges. Home health care agencies are one of the alternatives for assisting family members in caring for an aging family member (HelpageAsia, 2021).

A. **HOME HEALTH AGENCIES**

Home care refers to any professional support services that enable a person to live comfortably in their own home. In-home care services can help an aged person who needs help living independently, managing chronic health issues, recovering from a medical setback, or who has special needs or a handicap. Professional caregivers such as nurses, aides, and therapists provide short-term or long-term care in the home, depending on the individual's needs (The Care You Need in the Place You Love, n.d.).

Home care may be the key to achieving the highest quality of life possible. It can provide safety, security, and enhanced independence; it can help manage a chronic medical condition; it can help avoid unneeded hospitalization; and it can aid recovery after an illness, injury, or hospital stay—all while receiving care in the comfort and familiarity of one's own home (The Care You Need in the Place You Love, n.d.).

The following types of home care are available:

a. Help with daily activities such as dressing and bathing
b. Assistance with safely managing tasks around the house
c. Companionship
d. Therapy and rehabilitative services
e. Short- or long-term nursing care for an illness, disease, or disability—including tracheostomy and ventilator care

Types of Home Care Agencies

Not all home care agencies provide all of the listed services. Each home care agency is specifically designed to meet the requirements of the elderly and may provide services from one or more of the categories listed. While different types of home care meet different needs, they all aim to assist people live better, more independent lives while also offering support and peace of mind to their families.

1. ***Personal Care and Companionship.*** Non-medical care, home health aide services, senior care, homemaker care, assistive care, or companion care are all terms used to describe non-medical care. It facilitates freedom and safety by assisting with daily activities such as bathing and dressing, meal preparation, and home responsibilities.

   Personal Care and Companionship services may include:

   a. Assistance with self-care, such as grooming, bathing, dressing, and using the toilet
   b. Enabling safety at home by assisting with ambulation, transfer (e.g., from bed to wheelchair, wheelchair to toilet), and fall prevention

c. Assistance with meal planning and preparation, light housekeeping, laundry, errands, medication reminders, and escorting to appointments
   d. Companionship and engaging in hobbies and activities
   e. Supervision for someone with dementia or Alzheimer's disease

How Is Care Provided? Personal care and companionship do not require a doctor's prescription. Care is provided on an ongoing basis on a schedule that matches the needs of the client, up to 24 hours a day, seven days a week, with the option of live-in care.

2. **Private Duty Nursing Care.** Home-based skilled nursing, long-term nursing care, catastrophic care, tracheostomy care, ventilator care, nursing care, shift nursing, hourly nursing, or adult nursing are all terms used to describe home-based skilled nursing. Adults with a chronic disease, injury, or handicap get long-term, hourly nursing care at home.

<u>Private Duty Nursing Care services may include:</u>

   a. Care for diseases and conditions such as Traumatic brain injury (TBI), Spinal cord injury (SCI), ALS, MS
   b. Ventilator care
   c. Tracheostomy care
   d. Monitoring vital signs
   e. Administering medications
   f. Ostomy/gastrostomy care
   g. Feeding tube care
   h. Catheter care

How Is Care Provided? A doctor must write a prescription for private duty nursing care. Care is usually offered in shifts, which can last up to 24 hours a day, seven days a week.

3. **Home Health Care**. Medicare-certified home health care, intermittent skilled care, or visiting nurse services are other terms for the same thing. Short-term, physician-directed care aimed at helping patients avoid or recover from disease, injury, or hospitalization.

Home Health Care services may include:

a. Short-term nursing services
b. Physical therapy
c. Occupational therapy
d. Speech language pathology
e. Medical social work
f. Home health aide services

How Is Care Provided? A doctor's prescription is required for home health care. Visits from expert clinicians take up to an hour and are provided on a short-term basis until individual goals are reached.

B. ENTREPRENEURSHIP IN NURSING

Nurse entrepreneurs assist the creation of specialized products and services, upgraded technology, software, and safety measures to meet gaps in the current health-care delivery system.

A nurse entrepreneur, according to the International Council of Nurses (2004), is "a proprietor of a firm that offers nursing services of a direct care, educational, research, administrative, or consulting type." As a result, the nurse is self-employed and directly responsible to the client (individual, private, or public entity) for whom they provide services (Liu & D'Aunno, 2011). These nurses may have their own clinical practice, own a business (such as a nursing home or pharmaceutical company), or work as consultants in fields such as education or research. Nurse entrepreneurs are innovators who create incentives that lead to change, health system transformation, and leadership demonstration (Raine, 2003).

Nurse entrepreneurs can use their enterprises to produce and market medical products or devices, provide direct patient care or patient advocacy, educate or train other professionals or members of the community, or give health-related advice, among other things (ICN, 2004).

The application of creativity to develop a new idea, improve service or delivery techniques, or develop new products or new ways to use existing items is a basic element of entrepreneurship. At the very least, entrepreneurial nurses are advanced practice nurses who create products or services that they may market to external sources, combining these characteristics with advanced or specialty skills and knowledge.

Entrepreneurial Opportunities in Nursing

Nurses are becoming more entrepreneurial in the twenty-first century, and many are realizing that they may start small, medium, and large businesses at any stage in their careers (Press et al., 2021)

Nurse entrepreneurs can leverage their nursing education and business experience to launch new businesses in the healthcare field. They can help them build, promote, and run their own businesses. Some specialists can even apply their knowledge to the development of medical devices, computer systems, or home health goods (Press et al., 2021)

To set out as a Nurse Entrepreneur, some key skills are necessary:

a) Creativity
b) Business-oriented mindset,
c) Ability to find funding
d) Identifying a niche market
e) Establishing a consistent customer base

Services offered by Nurse Entrepreneurs

a) *Concierge Nursing* is a new sort of business concept in which an elderly patient hires a nurse directly for a fee. The traditional idea of concierge nursing is to accompany plastic surgery patients home following their procedure. Many of these patients have drains, several bandages, and are in a lot of discomfort when they leave the hospital. Having a concierge nurse at your bedside in your home or hotel provides comfort and help.

b) *Appointment Assistance.* Nurses volunteer to assist geriatric patients in getting to appointments. They aid them in selecting which care options are best for them. Some even stay at their patients' bedsides to provide support and counseling throughout the process.

c) *Healthcare Consulting.* Another option is to assist elderly patients in interpreting medical information. As a result, medical errors are reduced to a minimum. This may be especially valuable for elderly individuals who require complex, continuing care, such as for cancer.

d) *Wellness Coaching.* Patients who are elderly may require assistance in preserving their health. Nurses bring a unique perspective to health and wellbeing as health coaches because their understanding of medicine, disease, and health promotion, as well as real patient experiences, is unrivaled in the health coaching industry.

e) *Holistic Care.* Natural and holistic medical treatment are becoming increasingly popular. This type of company provides a one-of-a-kind strategy to treating specific conditions.

f) *Hospital Photography.* A nurse might desire to start a photography business to chronicle families' final moments of life, such as a picture shoot in hospice or with premature babies in the neonatal intensive care unit. This type of service would necessitate a nurse who is not only versed in the grieving process, but also recognizes that the photographs serves as a one-of-a-kind present for families.

g) *Hospice Care.* End-of-life care is still a highly sought-after service in and of itself. The nurse must be able to care for an old patient as well as their complete family. And the job entails interacting with patients who are nearing the end of their lives.

h) *Nurse Consulting.* A nurse might potentially start a business to assist healthcare workers in working with newly diagnosed cancer patients by utilizing medical metaphors to describe the type of cancer they have and what their next actions should be. This procedure aids patients and their families in comprehending the disease and, as a result, making informed treatment decisions (9 Great Business Ideas for Nurse Entrepreneurs - Small Business Trends, 2019).

Important components to become a nurse entrepreneur:

1. *Quality:* It's crucial to be a creative thinker who can turn a thought into a reality. As a foundation for being a nurse entrepreneur, a nurse entrepreneur must have expertise of management, including strategic planning, business plan development, marketing, management information systems, leadership, and financial management.

2. *Role:* Entrepreneur is defined as a person who can organize, manage, and deal with a business and is prepared to take chances in order to profit.

3. *Option and Success:* Nurses have a variety of choices for becoming entrepreneurs. Of course, these options are based on a foundation of skills and inventiveness, as well as nurse knowledge that may be improved to become a successful nurse (Kelompoksatune, 2001).

5 Steps to Becoming a Nursepreneur (Nurse Entrepreneur)):

1. *Assessment:* Assessing nurses' clinical abilities and expertise, as well as the market's (client/community) needs.

2. *Diagnosis:* Following the assessment, the next step is to determine the diagnosis. After determining the market's needs, the following phase in the business world is to map the potential into which we might enter to meet those wants. The stage diagnosis is the mapping of potential in this step.

3. *Plan:* Once we have determined the market potential, the following stage is to devise a strategy for breaking into the real market. We should have a clear and detailed business concept at this level of planning.

4. *Implementation:* This is a step toward action for us. A clear business concept must be translated into physical form. This is the most important stage in the process of doing business, and it is also the most challenging. Although everybody can have an idea, not everyone is willing to act on it.

5. *Evaluation:* The evaluation is a crucial aspect of any system and should not be overlooked. We can decide whether or not our plan was implemented successfully based on this assessment. In the corporate sector, the

evaluation will show us whether the notion we've implemented has been successful or not. If we are successful, we can make improvements, but if we are not, we can rethink our plans and strategy (Kelompoksatune, 2001).

SUMMARY: This chapter emphasized the importance of identifying best practices and skill sets transferable from direct caregiving to company leadership as more nurses move beyond the bedside to explore entrepreneurship. It also underlined the significance of understanding how nurses have changed their perspectives in order to make the adjustment, as well as the importance of self-care. It discussed the difficulties that nurse entrepreneurs face, as well as how entrepreneurship can help nurses have a greater impact, achieve greater career and life satisfaction, and feel more empowered by allowing them to pursue their personal vision and passion for improving health outcomes through innovative approaches.

> **Learning Activity:** Reflect on the following questions and answer as honestly as you can.
>
> 1. Would it be wrong to consider healthcare as a business?
> 2. Is business acumen necessary in becoming a healthcare professional?
> 3. How do you balance and harmonize healthcare as a business and as an altruistic service?
> 4. What is the importance of entrepreneurship and innovation in the healthcare industry?
> 5. What are the pros and cons of home care and home health agencies?

Guiding Question:

The students are expected to act as nurse entrepreneurs and develop a business plan around a specific service or system they have learned about under this chapter. The only requirement shall be that their target market should be geriatric and older adult patients. They should follow the five (5) steps of becoming a nurse entrepreneur as learned under this chapter. They shall submit their proposed completed business plan as their output.

Notes

Chapter 1
1. Brunner & Suddarth. (2007). Textbook of Medical-Surgical Nursing 11th ed., Lippincott Williams & Wilkins.
2. Central Intelligence Agency. (2016). The world fact book: Philippines. 2017.
3. Chenbaum, W. & Bengtson, V. *(1994). Re-engaging the Disengagement Theory of Aging: on the history and assessment of theory. Development in Gerontology.Gerontologist. 34(6): 756–763.*
4. Coscoluella, C., & Faustino, E. R. (2014). A legacy of public health (Tan C. I. Ed., 2nded.). Manila, Philippines: Department of Health.
5. Diggs J. (2008). Activity Theory of Aging. In: Loue S.J., Sajatovic M. (eds) Encyclopedia of Aging and Public Health. Springer, Boston.
6. Harman, D. (1956) Aging: a theory based on free radical and radiation chemistry. J Gerontol. 11 (3): 298–300.
7. Help Age Global Network. (2017a). Ageing and health: Philippines.
8. Jin K. Modern biological theories of ageing. Aging Dis. 2010; 1(2): 72–74.
9. Makofsky, N. (2012) How Does Caring for Aging Parents Affect Family Life? *Published Dec 6, 2012.* Retrieved on August 11, 2020 from: https://mom.com/kids/4870-how-does-caring-aging-parents-affect-family-life/
10. Thomas, K. & Segur M. (n.d.). Co-owners and directors of Hearts and Hands Counseling.
11. *Weinert, B. & Timiras P., (2003). Invited review: theories of aging. Appl Physiol.; 95:1706–1716.*
12. Zs.-Nagy, I. (1994). *The Membrane Hypothesis of Aging.* Florida: CRC Press.

Chapter 2
1. Adams, K. (2012). Planning for "Successful Aging" at Mid-life Retrieved on August 12, 2020 from https://www.psychologytoday.com/us/blog/mid-life-what-crisis/201210/planning-successful aging-mid-life
2. Bassem, E., & Higgins, K. (2011). *American Family Physician.* 1;83(1):48-56.
3. Brodaty, H. & Moore, C. M. (1997). The Clock Drawing Test for Dementia of the Alzheimer's Type: a comparison of three scoring methods in a memory disorders clinic. *International Journal of Geriatric Psychiatry*, 12, 619-627.
4. Chauhan, B. (n.d). 8 Tips for Succesful Aging. https://www.summitmedicalgroup.com/news/living-well/8-tips-successful-aging/
5. Inouye, S. K., van Dyck, C. H., Alessi, C. A., et al (1990) Clarifying confusion: the Confusion Assessment Method. *Annals of Internal Medicine*, 113, 941-948.
6. Folkman, S. & Lazarus, R. (1980) An analysis of coping in a middle aged community sample. *Journal of Health and Social Behaviour*, 21, 219-239.
7. Shulman, K., Shedletsky, R. & Silver, I. (1986). The challenge of time: clock drawing and cognitive function in the elderly. *International Journal of Geriatric Psychiatry*, 1, 135-140.

8. Rybolt, B. (2016). 8 Tips for Successful Aging. Summit medical Group. Retrieved onAugust 12, 2020 from https://www.summitmedicalgroup.com/news/living-well/8-tips-successful-aging/
9. Yesavage, J., Brink, T., Rose, T., *et al* (1983). Development and validation of a geriatric depression screening scale. *Journal of Psychiatric Research*, 17, 37-49

Chapter 3
1. Burggraf, V. (1980). Promoting Education; Improving quality in long-term care, *J Gerontol Nurs* 30(3):3, 2004
2. Ebersole, P., Hess, P, Touhy, T. & Jett, K. (2005). *Gerontological Nursing & Healthy Aging*, 2nd. Elsevier Mosby.
3. Gulanick, M. & Myers, J. (2016). *Nursing care Plans – E Book: Nursing Diagosis and Intervention* 9th ed. Elsevier Health Sciences/
4. 10 Early Signs and Symptoms of Alzheimer's from: https://www.alz.org/alzheimers-dementia/10_signs

Chapter 4
1. American Association of Colleges of Nursing (AACN) & The John A. Hartford Foundation Institute for Geriatric Nursing. (2000). Older Adults: Recommended Baccalaureate Competencies and Curricular Guidelines for Geriatric Nursing Care [pdf]. Retrieved July 28, 2009 from:
http://www.aacn.nche.edu/Education/pdf/Gercomp.pdf
2. Crandall, L.G., White, D.L., Schuldheis, S., & Talerico, K.A. (2009). Initiating Person-Centered Care Practices in Long-term Care Facilities. Journal of Gerontological Nursing, 2007, 33(11), 47-56.
3. Potter, P.A. & Perry, A.G. (2009). Canadian Fundamentals of Nursing (4rd eds.). Canada: Mosby Elsevier.
4. Saffron, D.G., Miller, W., & Beckman, H. Organizational dimensions of relationship-centered care theory, evidence, and practice. Journal of General Internal Medicine, 21 (1): 9-15.
5. Wiersman, E., & Dupuis, S. (2007). Managing responsive behaviors. Canadian Nursing Home, 18 (2): 17-22.

Chapter 5
1. Advanced Directives. Retrieved on August 16, 2020 from https://www.makatimed.net.ph/patient-and-visitor-guide/patient-references/advanced-directives
2. Beth, L. (n.d.). Ethical Caregiving and Protecting Elders. Retrieved on August 16, 2020 from: https://www.asaging.org/blog/ethical-caregiving-and-protecting-elders
3. Cifu, D., Lew, H. & Oh-Park, M. (2019). Geriatric Rehabilitation. Elsevier Inc. https://doi.org/10.1016/C2016-0-04564-3
4. Code of Ethics Review Group, New Zealand Psychological Society, the New Zealand College of Clinical Psychologists and the New Zealand Psychologists Board. Code of Ethics for Psychologists in Aotearoa/New Zealand 2002 [Internet]. [cited 2015 Oct. 20]; Available from:
http://www.psychologistsboard.org.nz/cms_show_download.php?id=237

5. Feder, J., Komisar, HL., & Niefeld, M. (2000). Long-term care in the United States: an overview. Health Affairs. 19(3):40–56.
6. Harris, et. al. (2000). National Council on the Aging
7. Jacobs, S. (n.d.). Ethical Issues in the Health Care of Older People. Oklahoma State University. Retrieved on August 17, 2020 from: https://www.researchgate.net/publication/287206274_Ethical_Issues_in_the_Health_Care_of_Older_People
8. Kane, R., Ouslander, J., Abrass, I. & Resnick, B. (2013). Essentials of Clinical Geriatrics, Seventh Edition. McGraww-Hill Education LLC.
9. Maher, R. L., Hanlon, J., & Hajjar, E. R. (2014). Clinical consequences of polypharmacy in elderly. *Expert opinion on drug safety, 13*(1), 57–65. https://doi.org/10.1517/14740338.2013.827660
10. Moberg, O. (1971). Spiritual well-being. White press Conference on Aging. Washington DC. Retrieved on August 17, 2020 from https://files.eric.ed.gov/fulltext/ED057348.pdf
11. Moberg, O. (2001). Aging and spirituality. New York: Haworth.
12. Providing Care and Comfort at the End of Life. Retrieved on August 16, 2020 from: https://www.nia.nih.gov/health/providing-comfort-end-life
13. What Is Palliative Care? Retrieved on August 16, 2020 from https://getpalliativecare.org/whatis/

Chapter 6
1. Smith, M. (2006). "Getting the Facts: Communicating with the Elderly," The Geriatric Mental Health Training Series, for the Hartford Center of Geriatric Nursing Excellence, College of Nursing, University of Iowa.
2. https://nursekey.com/communicating-with-older-adults/

Chapter 7
1. Nurseslabs. (2013, June 8). Documentation & Reporting In Nursing - Nurseslabs. https://nurseslabs.com/documentation-reporting-in-nursing/.
2. http://compliantlearningresources.com.au/network/lotus/files/2016/06/Documenting-Skills-in-Aged-Care-Progress-Notes.pdf
3. http://compliantlearningresources.com.au/network/lotus/files/2016/06/Documenting-Skills-in-Aged-Care-Progress-Notes.pdf

Chapter 8
1. Gitlin LN, Wolff J. Family involvement in care transitions of older adults: What do we know and where do we go from here? Annual Review of Gerontology and Geriatrics. 2012;31(1):31–64.
2. National: NIH Publication-2030 Problems on Caring for Aging Baby Boomers. Ageing, Older Persons And The 2030 Agenda For Sustainable Development. Retrieved From: https://www.ncbi.nlm.nih.gov/pmc/articles/PMC1464018/#:~:text=The%20%E2%

3. Badana A. and Andel R. (2018). Aging in the Philippines. *The Gerontologist*, Volume 58, Issue 2, April 2018, Pages 212-218, https://doi.org/10.1093/geront/gn
4. Bakerjian D (2020). Overview of Geriatric Care. https://www.msdmanuals.com/professional/geriatrics/providing-care-to-older-adults/overview-of-geriatric-care
5. Johns Hopkins Medicine. (2021, January 1). Specialists in Aging: Do You Need a Geriatrician? | Johns Hopkins Medicine. https://www.hopkinsmedicine.org/health/wellness-and-prevention/specialists-in-aging-do-you-need-a-geriatrician.
6. Best Master of Science in Nursing Degrees (2015, October 30). What Is a Gerontology Nurse?. | Find a Master of Science in Nursing Program. https://www.bestmasterofscienceinnursing.com/faq/what-is-a-gerontology-nurse/.
7. Regis College. (n.d.). What Does an Occupational Therapist Do? Roles And Responsibilities. https://www.regiscollege.edu/blog/occupational-therapy/what-does-occupational-therapist-do-roles-and-responsibilities.
8. What Is a Physical Therapist?. (2020, July 12). What is a physical therapist?. https://www.kumc.edu/school-of-health-professions/physical-therapy-rehabilitation-science-and-athletic-training/doctor-of-physical-therapy/what-is-a-physical-therapist.html.
9. Aged Care News. (n.d.). Aged Care news. https://healthtimes.com.au/hub/aged-care/2/news/nm/speech-pathology-should-be-routinely-offered-in-aged-care-facilities-says.
10. Case Management Services. (n.d.). Case Management Services. http://www.caregiverresourcecenter.com/counseling_services.htm.
11. Healthcare Basics. (n.d.). What Is an Interdisciplinary Team? | Sharecare. https://www.sharecare.com/health/health-care-basics/what-is-interdisciplinary-team.

Chapter 9

1. Sandeen, C. (2008). Boomers, Xers, and Millennials: Who are They and What Do They Really Want from Continuing Higher Education? *Continuing Higher education review*, Vol. 72, 2008 https://files.eric.ed.gov/fulltext/EJ903434.pdf
2. Baby Boomers, Retirement and Real Estate. (n.d.). Baby Boomers, Retirement and Real Estate. https://pinnacle.ph/research/baby-boomers-retirement-real-estate.
3. Lucentales Ruel G. (n.d). The Philippine response to the challenges of ageing. *From:*https://www.mhlw.go.jp/bunya/kokusaigyomu/asean/asean/kokusai/siryou/dl/h16_philippines2.pdf
4. HelpAge International. (n.d.). Sustainable Development Goals | What We Do |. https://www.helpage.org/what-we-do/post2015-process/.
5. United Nations (n.d.). International Day Of Older Persons https://www.un.org/en/observances/older-persons-day.
6. United Nations (2021.). Events | United Nations. United Nations. https://www.un.org/en/events/pastevents/pdfs/Madrid.
7. The National Academies Press. (n.d.). Extending Life, Enhancing Life: A National Research Agenda on Aging | The National Academies Press. https://www.nap.edu/read/1632/chapter/3.
8. Badana, A. N., & Andel, R. (2018, April 1). Aging In the Philippines | The Gerontologist | Oxford Academic. OUP Academic. https://academic.oup.com/gerontologist/article/58/2/212/4792953.

Chapter 10
1. Barnes J., (2020). How to Become an Advocate for the Elderly https://www.wikihow.com/Become-an-Advocate-for-the-Elderly
2. WHO (2017) Mental health of older adults https://www.who.int/news-room/fact-sheets/detail/mental-health-of-older-adults
3. Home Health Care. (n.d.). Home Health Care. https://eldercare.acl.gov/public/resources/factsheets/home_health_care.aspx.
4. Johns Hopkins Medicine. (2021, January 1). Types of Home Health Care Services | Johns Hopkins Medicine. https://www.hopkinsmedicine.org/health/caregiving/types-of-home-health-care-services.
5. National Institute on Aging (2021, May 14). What Are Palliative Care And Hospice Care?.. https://www.nia.nih.gov/health/what-are-palliative-care-and-hospice-care.
6. HelpGuide.org. (2020, December 1). Adult Day Care Services - HelpGuide.org. https://www.helpguide.org/articles/senior-housing/adult-day-care-services.htm.
7. SeniorLiving.org. (2019, December 12). Retirement Homes for Seniors | Are There Retirement Homes Near Me?. https://www.seniorliving.org/retirement/homes/.

Chapter 11
1. New Homepage. (2021). HelpAge International. https://www.helpage.org/silo/files/advocacy-with-older-people-some-practical-suggestions.
2. WikiHow. (2021, September 9). 4 Ways To Become an Advocate for the Elderly - https://www.wikihow.com/Become-an-Advocate-for-the-Elderly.
3. Mental Health Of Older Adults. (2017, December 12). Mental health of older adults. https://www.who.int/news-room/fact-sheets/detail/mental-health-of-older-adults.

Chapter 12
1. Anderson J., (2013). The Importance of Grandparents. https://www.aplaceformom.com/blog/10-22-13-reasons-grandparents-matter-more-than-ever/
2. 10 Reasons Grandparents Matter More Than Ever. (n.d.). A Place for Mom. https://www.aplaceformom.com/caregiver-resources/articles/grandparents-matter-more-than-ever.

Chapter 13
1. Patdu I. and Tenorio Allan S. (2016). Establishing the Legal Framework of Telehealth in the Philippines. ACTA MEDICA PHILIPPINA 2 VOL. 50 NO. 4 2016 From: https://actamedicaphilippina.upm.edu.ph
2. Cranford, L. (2020, May 1). *Telemedicine Vs. Telehealth: What's the Difference?.* Chiron Health. https://chironhealth.com/blog/telemedicine-vs-telehealth-whats-the-difference/.
3. Foster M., (2014). Facilitators and Barriers to the Adoption of Telehealth in Older Adults. CIN: Computers, Informatics, Nursing & Vol. 32, No. 11, 523–533. From: https://nursing.ceconnection.com/ovidfiles/00024665-201411000-00003.pdf

Chapter 14

1. International Council of Nurses (2004). Guidelines on the nurse entre/intrapreneur providing nursing service. Geneva, Switzerland; 2004. https://ipnig.com/education/Guidelines-NurseEntre-ICN.pdf
2. HelpageAsia, (2019). *Ageing Population In the Philippines | HelpAge Asia.* HelpAge Asia. https://ageingasia.org/ageing-population-philippines/.
3. The Care You Need In the Place You Love. (n.d.). BAYADA Home Health Care. https://www.bayada.com/homehealthcare/what-is-homecare/.
4. Press, D., Vannucci, M. J., & Weinstein, S. M. (n.d.). The Nurse Entrepreneur: Empowerment Needs, Challenges, And Self-care P | NRR. The nurse entrepreneur: empowerment needs, challenges, and self-care p | NRR. https://www.dovepress.com/the-nurse-entrepreneur-empowerment-needs-challenges-and-self-care-prac-peer-reviewed-fulltext-article-NRR.
5. 9 Great Business Ideas for Nurse Entrepreneurs - Small Business Trends. (2019, July 10). Small Business Trends. https://smallbiztrends.com/2019/07/nurse-entrepreneur-business-ideas.html.
6. Kelompoksatune (2001, December 24). Nursepreneur – Relation of Nursing Concept With Entrepreneurship. Relation of Nursing Concept with Entrepreneurship. https://nursepreneurbestfkepunpad.wordpress.com/tag/nursepreneur/.

www.ingramcontent.com/pod-product-compliance
Lightning Source LLC
Chambersburg PA
CBHW081001170526
45158CB00010B/2869